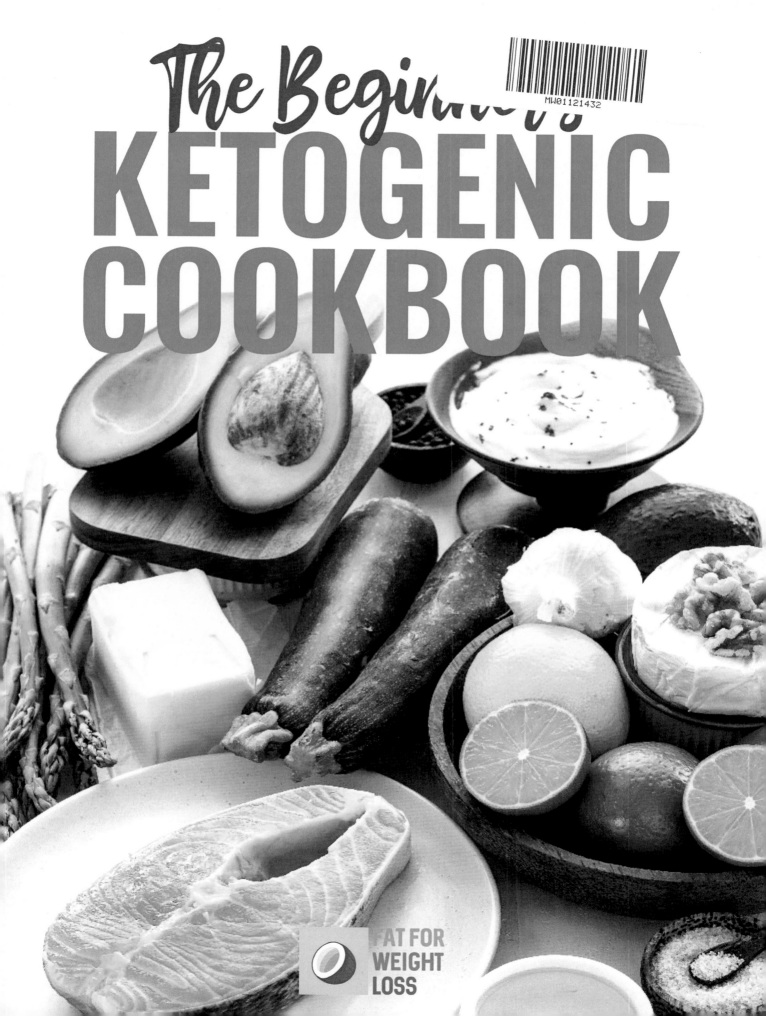

The Beginner's
KETOGENIC
COOKBOOK

FAT FOR
WEIGHT
LOSS

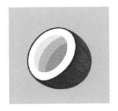

FATFORWEIGHTLOSS

UK | USA | CANADA | IRELAND | AUSTRALIA
INDIA | NEW ZEALAND | SOUTH AFRICA

Published by Aaron Day, 2018

· · ·

· · ·

ISBN-13: 978-1725954489
ISBN-10: 1725954486

· · ·

www.fatforweightloss.com.au

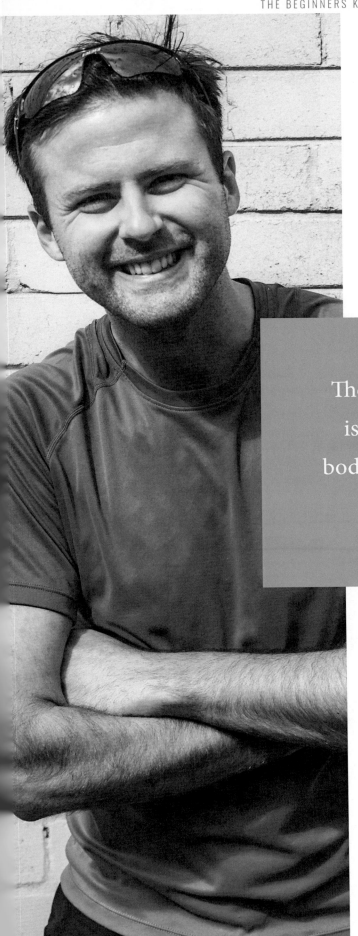

INTRODUCTION

You might not believe that weight loss without exercise is possible. You probably don't believe it's possible to improve your current exercise performance levels. You think it's impossible to build muscle whilst restricting carbohydrates, and most of all, you don't believe increasing your fat intake could ever be healthy.

You've probably heard about the ketogenic diet, but if you haven't, I'm going to explain it in very simple terms.

The basic idea of the ketogenic diet is focused on enabling your own body to turn to fat for energy instead of carbohydrates, or protein.

There are many benefits to eating a ketogenic diet, including elimination of many common diseases such as epilepsy, diabetes, polycystic ovary syndrome (PCOS), irritable bowel syndrome (IBS), GERD, heartburn and non-alcoholic fatty liver disease (NAFLD).

The main concept of ketogenic weight loss is to help you be in a state of caloric restriction without maintaining the sufficient calories and being hungry. Your body just burns its own fat as it needs to.

Excess carbohydrates turn to fat in the body anyway, so doesn't it make sense to train your body to burn fat if you want to lose fat?

WHY SHOULD YOU GO KETO?

So why would we want to reduce the amount of sugar we consume and switch our bodies over to burn fat instead?

 Metabolically, fat is a superior fuel for the body

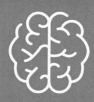 Consuming fats enhances your brain function and gives mental stability

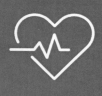 Greater health and longevity that comes from controlling your blood sugar levels naturally

Ketones (produced by burning fat) are the preferred fuel source for vital organs such as the muscles, heart, liver, and brain. Let's look at some of the other benefits to nutritional ketosis:

• Natural hunger control
• Lowered inflammation levels
• Normalised metabolic function
• Lowered blood pressure

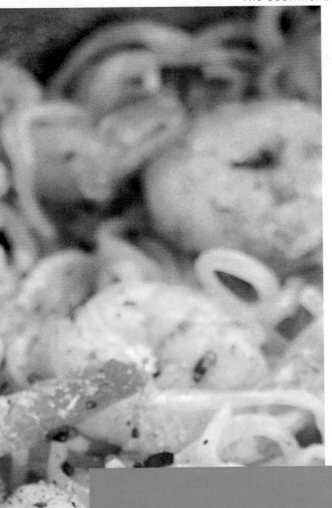

- Mental clarity
- Effortless weight loss
- Reduced triglycerides
- Lowered levels of LDL particles (*bad cholesterol*)
- Increased levels of HDL particles (*good cholesterol*)
- Increased sex drive
- Better fertility
- Eliminated heartburn
- Improved immune system
- Slowing the aging process
- Reduced acne breakouts
- Faster recovery from exercise
- Decreased anxiety and mood swings
- ……we could go on and on!

Not only does nutritional ketosis benefit the body, weight issues also respond extremely well to the approach.

A study by Harvard School of Public Health analysed 53 studies involving 67,000 dieters and found that those who cut back on carbs were two and a half pounds lighter after a year than those who embraced a "low fat" approach.

For decades, there has been debate over the merits of a low-fat diet, which was endorsed as the best route to weight loss in the 1970s. Now, major research published in The Lancet Diabetes & Endocrinology, back a low carbohydrate approach as a more effective diet.

HISTORY OF THE KETOGENIC DIET

One of the most misunderstood concepts in history is this one - fat makes you fat. Does this logic apply to, for instance, going green after eating too many cucumbers? Of course not! Fat will make you fat only when it is paired with excess carbohydrates.

All the studies that say fat causes heart disease link back to one study, and it's the reason why we think saturated fat causes heart disease. It was developed in the early 1950s by Ancel Benjamin Keys.

In his lab, Keys ran experiments looking for early indications of disease. What you must remember is that in the 1950's, no health issue seemed more urgent than heart disease.

Keys' most famous findings were contained in the Seven Countries Study, which showed that the risk and rates of heart attack and stroke cardiovascular risk, both at the population level and the individual level, were directly correlated to the level of total serum cholesterol.

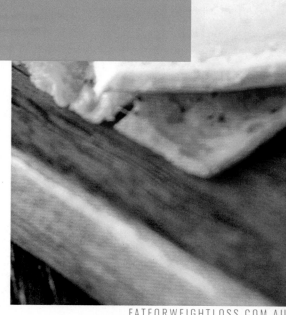

It demonstrated that the association between blood cholesterol level and coronary heart disease (CHD) risk from 5 to 40 years' follow-up is found consistently across different cultures.

Even before the study had begun, its methods had been criticised. Jacob Yerushalmy and Herman E. Hilleboe pointed out that, for an earlier study demonstrating this association, Keys had selected six countries out of 21 for which data were available.

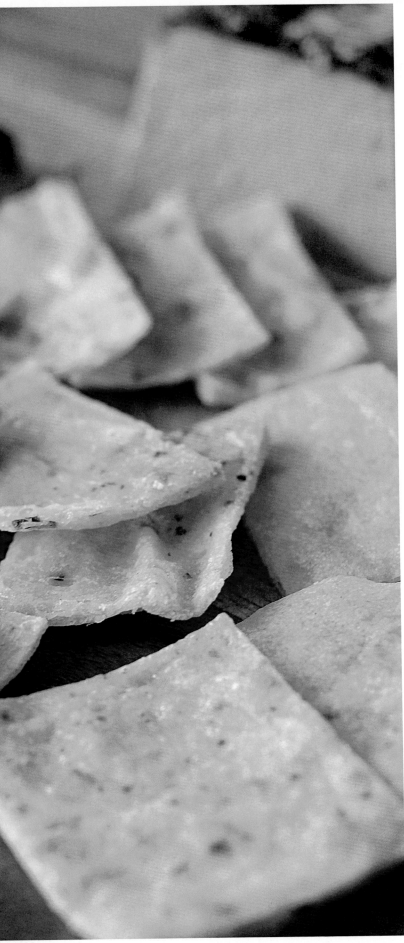

Analysis of the full dataset made the analysis of fat intake and heart disease unclear. Because of this, the association between the percentage of fat calories and mortality from heart disease was not valid.

It wasn't until 2014 when Nina Teicholz (author of "The Big Fat Surprise") reviewed the study, and in doing so found that one country, Crete, whose results formed the majority of the evidence from the study, was conducted during Lent, thereby causing Keys to dramatically undercount the amount of saturated fat eaten.

CORRELATION VS CAUSATION

EXAMPLE 1

The faster windmills are observed to rotate; the more wind there is observed to be. Therefore, wind is caused by the rotation of windmills. (or, simply put: windmills, as their name indicates, are machines used to produce wind.)

EXAMPLE 2

As ice cream sales increase, the rate of drowning deaths increases sharply. Therefore, ice cream consumption causes drowning.

EXAMPLE 3

Since the 1950s, both the atmospheric CO_2 level and obesity levels have increased sharply. Hence, atmospheric CO_2 causes obesity.

HOW TO START THE KETOGENIC DIET

"What advice would you give to a beginner?"

As a beginner, it's helpful to gain information from other people who have already started the ketogenic diet. Whilst I'm here to guide you, I've also solicited the help of others by putting together the various advice I've received throughout my own journey.

I've compiled these responses into a list, then ordered the topics by popularity. The result is the best advice from people just like you, who have already started the ketogenic diet:

SIMPLICITY
Keep it simple!

ELECTROLYTES
Salt, magnesium and potassium

NUTRITION
Real food doesn't have ingredients, it is ingredients

PERSISTENCE
Just get through that first week

SCIENCE
Have a brief understanding on how the ketogenic diet works.

 Watch the video for complete explanation of these points

By now, you should have a simple grasp on how to start the ketogenic diet, but for a more in-depth explanation on how to start the ketogenic diet the right way the first time, read on!

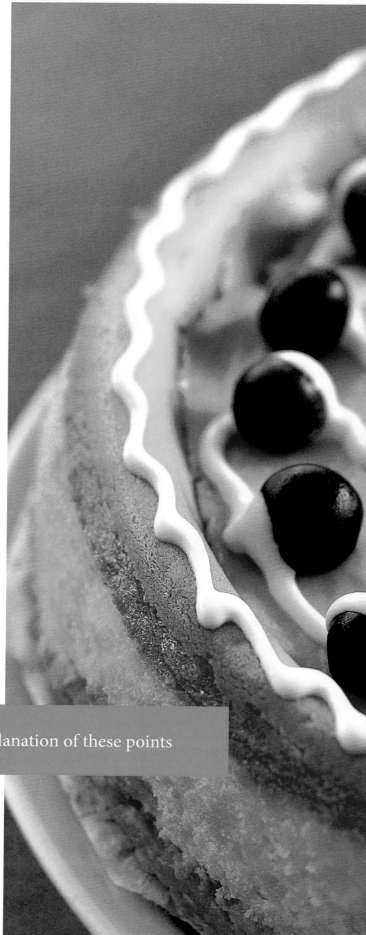

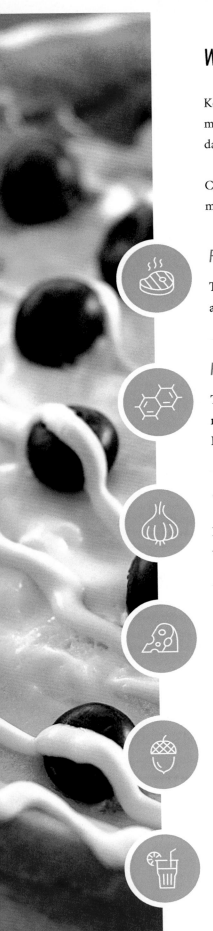

WHAT CAN I EAT ON THE KETOGENIC DIET?

Ketogenic diets can be different for everyone. Eat dark green leafy vegetables, fatty red meats, chicken with the skin left on, fish, offal (organ meat), eggs, seeds & nuts, full-fat dairy, or anything else rich in nutrition, fat, protein and fibre.

Carbs are a limit. Protein is a target. Fat is to be consumed to remove hunger and meet macros requirements.

FATS & OILS

Try to get your fat from natural sources like meat and nuts. Supplement with saturated and monounsaturated fats like coconut oil, butter, and olive oil.

PROTEIN

Try to stick with organic, pasture-raised and grass-fed meat where possible. Most meats don't have added sugar in them, so they can be consumed in moderate quantity. Remember that too much protein on a ketogenic diet is not a good thing.

VEGETABLES

Fresh is preferred, but frozen works too. Stick with above ground vegetables, leaning toward leafy/green options.

DAIRY

Most dairy is fine apart from milk. Make sure to buy full-fat dairy items. Harder cheeses typically have fewer carbs.

NUTS & SEEDS

In moderation, nuts and seeds can be used to create some fantastic textures. Try to use fattier nuts like macadamias and almonds.

BEVERAGES

Stay simple and stick to mostly water. You can flavour it if needed with stevia-based flavourings or lemon/lime juice.

MACRONUTRIENTS EXPLAINED

The main building blocks of food are carbohydrates, proteins, and fats. These are called macro nutrients. Just remember, macro means big, and micro means small.

Every piece of food is made up of a ratio of these building blocks. For example, chicken breast is high in protein, and pasta is high in carbohydrates.

Currently, most people eat a standard diet containing around 20% fats, 30% protein and 50% carbohydrates. It can be hard to venture outside of these well-known macro ratios.

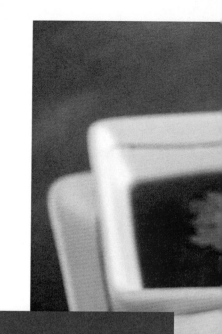

The ketogenic diet simply changes the ratio of these macronutrients. By limiting carbohydrates, moderating protein and increasing your total healthy fat intake, you put your body into a state of "ketosis." Instead of burning sugar and glucose for energy, your body starts to burn "ketones," which is an energy source that your body creates from fat.

Your body prefers burning fat for energy and it is the preferred source in your brain and muscles. It also has some remarkably positive results for many common chronic illnesses today.

Unfortunately, the general public haven't necessarily been exposed to the truth about nutritional ketosis, and therefore don't believe that it's a healthy state to be in.

Just as cholesterol was falsely labelled as a culprit for heart disease, ketones have been labelled as some kind of strange substance that you should avoid at all costs. This is simply not the case.

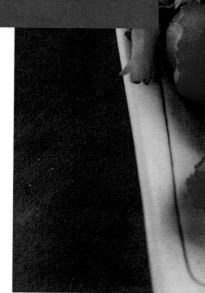

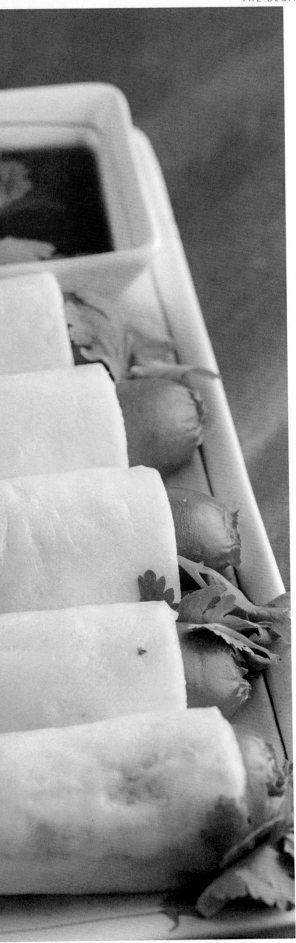

Your body will become what is called "fat adapted" whilst you re-teach it to use the stored fat as energy, all without feeling any starvation or typical diet hunger issues.

WHAT ARE THE DIFFERENT TYPES OF FAT THAT I CAN EAT?

Recommended fats to eat are **olive oil**, **grass-fed butter**, and **coconut oil**. There are actually four main types of fats. These are:

TRANS FATS

The most important fat to AVOID is Trans Fats. These types of fats have been chemically altered and industrially produced to improve their physical appearance and taste. This method, however, has been shown to significantly increase LDL cholesterol in humans (the bad one) by about 10% and has no impact on the protective HDL cholesterol.

Trans fat is a variant of unsaturated fat. 50 years ago, saturated fats were thought to be the enemy, as they were incorrectly linked with certain diseases. When trans fats were first introduced to food production, they were considered miraculous because they allowed a liquid oil to be converted to a solid spread without the "*adverse effects*" of saturated fat on blood cholesterol.

By 1990, research by Mensink and Katan showed trans fats elevated the harmful LDL cholesterol by about a tenth more than regular unsaturated fat. Compared with other fats, trans fats didn't have the benefit of elevating the protective HDL cholesterol. Mensink and Katan concluded that trans fats were the worst type of food that contributed to heart disease.

This was shown convincingly by Walter Willett in his 1993 study of US nurses. Those who reported eating a large number of trans fats (more than 5.7 grams a day) were around two-thirds more likely to have a heart attack than nurses eating less than 2.4 grams a day.

Trans fats from dairy and beef fat ("natural" trans) were not linked to heart disease risk.

SATURATED FATS (EAT MEAT, DAIRY)

Saturated fats are usually a solid at room temperature and oxidize slowly. They have a stable composition, which is why they are solid. This type of fat is most often found in animal foods including:

• Meat
• Dairy products

MONOUNSATURATED FAT (EAT AVOCADOS, OLIVE OIL, CASHEWS)

Monounsaturated fats are usually a liquid at room temperature. They have a weak composition which is why they convert to liquid easily. Monounsaturated fats are most often found in:

• Avocados
• Olives
• Almonds and cashews
• Olive oil and sesame oil

POLYUNSATURATED FAT (SUNFLOWER OIL, CORN OIL, SOYBEAN OIL, OMEGA 3, OMEGA 6)

Polyunsaturated fats can be tricky. This type of fat is mostly found in the following foods:

• Sunflower seeds and pumpkin seeds
• Corn oil, safflower oil, and soybean oil
• Pine nuts and walnuts

There is also a specific type of polyunsaturated fat called Omega 3 Fats, studied due to their significant effect on heart health and ability to lower triglyceride levels and increase high-density lipoproteins. This type of fat is best balanced with omega 6 fats at a ratio of 1:1, but you won't have to worry about that as long as you are eating whole foods. These particular fats can be found in the following:

• Fatty fish – including salmon, mackerel, herring, and tuna
• Certain seeds – including flax seeds and chia seeds
• Walnuts
• Algae

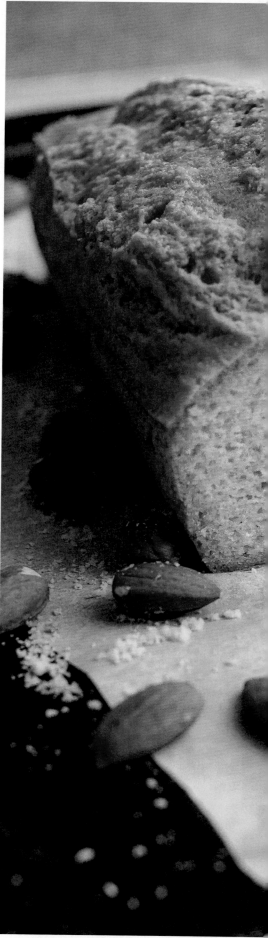

DO I HAVE TO EAT COCONUT OIL / MCT OIL?

Medium Chain Triglyceride (MCT) is a special type of saturated fat converted straight into energy by your liver and cannot be stored as fat.

The energy boosts you get from MCT oil is similar to carbs and is important to help you switch over to fat burning as easily as possible.

Coconut contains just over 60% MCT, so it's a beneficial way to get energy from a high-fat diet. MCT oil in particular has made a huge difference for me, especially when I tried the high-intensity cardio exercise on a keto diet, but mostly to keep my energy levels at an optimum level.

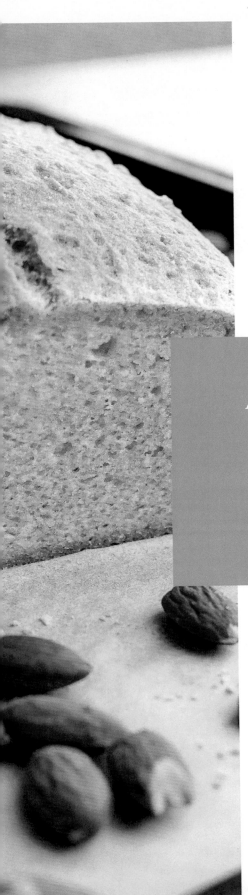

According to Dr. Laurie Cullen at the Women's Institute, when MCTs are absorbed into the bloodstream, they bypass the digestion process that longer chain fats go through.

MCT's provide quick energy for the body and are thus less likely to be stored in the fat cells. Further, Dr. Cullen says when a meal includes medium chain triglycerides, there is a significant increase in the amount of calories burned (thermogenic effect). When more calories are used, fewer are stored as fat, which helps reduce body fat levels.

Many keto diets and MCT oil spokespeople say MCT's energy sustaining powers can be explained as follows: when MCT oil is metabolized in the body, it behaves more like a carbohydrate energy source than a fat.

Remember, your current fuel preference for the body is carbohydrate (until you become fat adapted). Unlike other fats, MCT oil does not go through the lymphatic system. Instead, it is transported directly to the liver where it is metabolized so it releases energy like a carbohydrate and creates significant ketones (which can be used for fuel) in the process.

HOW MANY CARBOHYDRATES CAN YOU EAT ON THE KETOGENIC DIET?

Strictly speaking, the simple rule that most people follow is under 20 carbohydrates per day. What does that look like?

2 slices of bread is equal 20g of carbohydrates

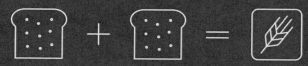

Usually, foods that contain carbohydrates also contain fibre. Because fibre doesn't contain any of the nasty aspects that carbohydrates do (simply speaking), we can safely eliminate them from the total amount of carbohydrates that we consume.

Your body will always attempt to use carbohydrates as a source of energy because they are so easily broken down into sugar in your body. This doesn't mean, however, that your body runs well on this fuel.

If you pull into a gas station, there is always a couple of different types of fuel you can choose to fill up with.

Carbohydrates are like the cheapest, dirtiest fuel, whilst fats are similar to the premium fuel. The cheap fuel will still get you to your destination, but it's filling your car with issues that you will have to pay for in the future.

Your body prefers running on healthy fats because they cause less inflammation, are longer lasting, and you can store the fuel easily on your body. Carbohydrates have to be turned into fat to be stored and will only be used when there is a lack of carbohydrates available.

Net Carbs Explained:

Total Carbohydrate	12g	4%
Dietary Fiber	4g	15%
Sugars	6g	

Net carbs = Total Carbs (including suger) - Fiber (12g Total Carbs) (6g of which is suger) - 4g (Fiber) = 8g Net Carbs

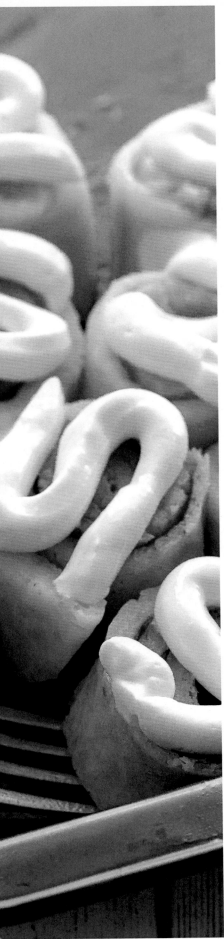

LAZY KETO IS SIMPLY LIMITING THE NUMBER OF CARBOHYDRATES YOU EAT

A keto diet is just a low carb diet coupled with a higher fat intake. The amount of carbs depends on each person, but it usually below 50 grams of net carbs per day. If you eat 10 grams of carbs, but that contains 5 grams of fibre, you will have consumed 5 grams of net carbs.

This limited amount of carbohydrate intake will switch your body over to burning ketones as your primary source of fuel. Alternatively, you can look at your body switching from being a sugar burning steam train with all the dirty black soot covering the engine, to a clean burning Tesla that runs on fat and ultimately does less damage to your body.

Keto diets are low in carbohydrates. This means you should avoid the following foods:

- Bread
- Pasta
- Sugar
- Milk
- Corn
- Beans
- Rice*
- Fruit*

*Unless you are refueling from exercise – still limit these.

What most people don't understand is that this is a normal metabolic state. When babies are born, they will go into a state of nutritional ketosis, relying on their mother's breast milk, which provides 25% energy from ketones. If you have ever skipped breakfast, you would most certainly have been in a state of Ketosis.

WON'T I BECOME TIRED IF I CUT OUT THE CARBS?

Carbs do equal energy, but like sugar, they only last for a limited amount of time. There is a by-product of fat consumption which is called Ketones.

In a state of carbohydrate depletion, ketones are used in your body as energy, particularly in the brain. Put simply, burning fat whilst being in a low carb state, also equals energy! And much more of it.

The Keto Diet can make you feel much more alert because your brain is getting much more energy from ketones than it ever did from carbohydrates.

WHAT OTHER CONDITIONS WILL A KETO DIET HELP?

There is a great amount of science-based evidence showing that the following conditions can be reversed or greatly improved on a keto diet.

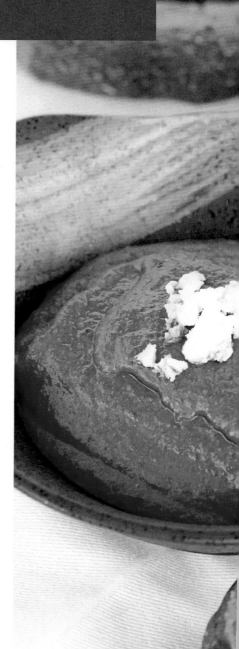

A keto diet has been used for many years to treat epilepsy. By stabilizing energy production and increasing blood ketone levels, the body is able to control seizures.

Blood ketone levels are also showing strong signs in the treatments of certain disorders such as Autism, ALS, Parkinson's disease and MS.

We know that aging is a result of the destruction of the human body, but you might not be aware that inflammation can accelerate aging. A keto diet can reduce inflammation significantly, therefore preventing the aging process.

Endurance athletes may be surprised to know that a keto diet can help with mitochondrial support, as it increases oxygen uptake and increases the efficiency of the mitochondrial biomechanics. This, in turn, can help in diseases such as Glucose Transporter Type 1 Deficiency, McArdle's Disease, and Pyruvate Dehydrogenase Complex Deficiency.

DIABETES AND INGESTING FAT

Type 2 Diabetes is one of the most avoidable diseases in the western world, and it has become an epidemic. Most of our population just don't understand what causes this disease.

People with diabetes are not affected most by large amounts of fat or protein. Insulin resistance is the key cause, and guess what causes insulin resistance; taking a ride on the carbohydrate roller coaster every 3-4 hours which eventually leads to insulin resistance, along with other factors.

When a person with diabetes eats a burger and fries, it's the carbohydrate one that sends their blood glucose spiraling out of control, not the meat and cheese. Fat is not to blame at all, it just happens to take the fall.

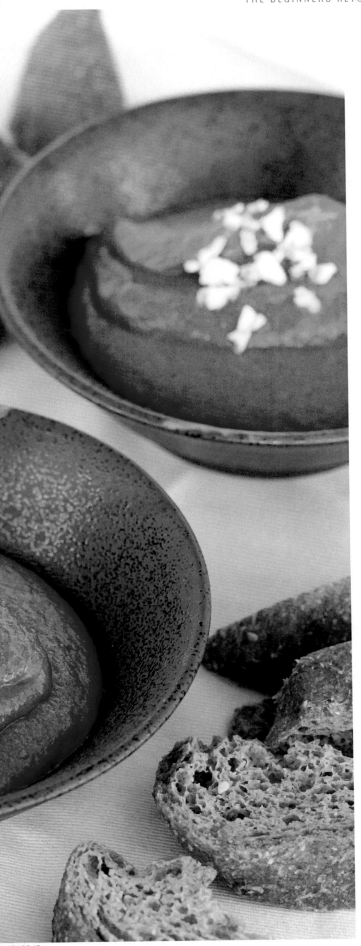

WHAT IS INSULIN RESISTANCE?

Before we talk about insulin resistance, let's talk about insulin. Insulin is made by your pancreas and allows your body to use glucose (sugar) from carbohydrates in your diet.

This particular molecule helps keep your blood sugar levels from getting too high (hyperglycemia) or too low (hypoglycemia).

A good way to remember this is that HYPER comes from too much sugar, and HYPO comes from not enough.

Your body regulates the amount of blood sugar in the blood by insulin. When the body has too much excess insulin, it can become insulin resistant. This has the ability to cause a multitude of other chronic health risks, including PCOS (For women) and Fatty Liver Disease.

CHOLESTEROL AND THE KETO DIET

Cholesterol plays an important role in our survival. The liver is careful to ensure the body always has enough, creating around 1000 – 1400 milligrams of it each day. The liver also has important feedback mechanisms that regulate how much it needs to produce from how much we get from our diet.

Cholesterol's main job is to insulate parts of our cells, build and maintain cell membranes, help digest fat soluble vitamins like Vitamin D (sun), E (skin), A (eyesight) and K (blood clotting) whilst also kick-starting many of the body's own pathways to producing hormones, including sex hormones!

Cardiac risk factors improve when blood sugar and insulin levels are lowered via dietary changes. HDL cholesterol goes up on a low carb, high-fat diet and triglycerides fall dramatically.

EATING A HIGH CHOLESTEROL DIET DOES NOT INCREASE HEART DISEASE

The American Journal of Clinical Nutrition undertook a study proving that eating a high-cholesterol diet does not increase the risk of heart disease.

The study followed 1,032 initially healthy men aged 42 to 60. The men consumed an average of about 2,800 milligrams of cholesterol a week; more than a quarter of it from eating an average of four eggs weekly. (An egg contains about 180 milligrams of cholesterol.)

After controlling for age, education, smoking, B.M.I., diabetes, hypertension, and other characteristics, the researchers found no association between cardiovascular disease and total cholesterol or egg consumption. The researchers also examined carotid artery thickness, a measure of atherosclerosis. They found no association between cholesterol consumption and artery thickness, either.

In Europe, countries that consume the most Saturated Fat have the Lowest Risk of Heart Disease

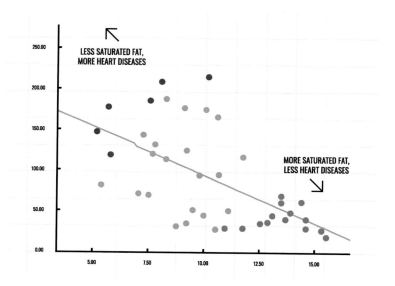

X: Total energy from saturated fat (%) | **Y:** Male age-standardised CHD deaths per 100,000
Figure 1: Saturated fat intake and CHD mortality in Europe (1998). R^2 Linear=0.339.

● **Countries with more heart diseases** | ● **Countries with less heart diseases**

● Belarus	● Denmark	● Ireland	● Finland
● Kazakhstan	● France	● United	● Iceland
● Ukraine	● Finland	● Kingdom	
● Azerbaijan	● Austria	● Norway	
● Georgia	● Switzerland	● Italy	
● Moldova	● Germany	● Spain	

Data from: Hoenselaar R. Further response from Hoenselaar. British Journal of Nutrition, 2012.

The Obesity Epidemic in the USA started at almost the exact same time the **Low-Fat Dietary Guidelines** were Published.

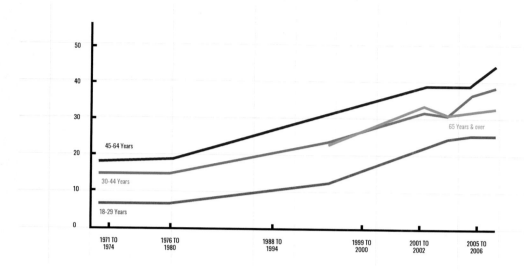

X: Year | **Y:** Percent

Source: National Centre for Health Statistics (US). Health, United States, 2008: With Special Feature on the Health of Young Adults. Hyattsville (MD): National Centre for Health Statistics (US); 2009 Mar. Chartbook.

The Diseases of Civilization Increased as Butter and Lard were Replaced with Vegetable Oils and Trans Fats

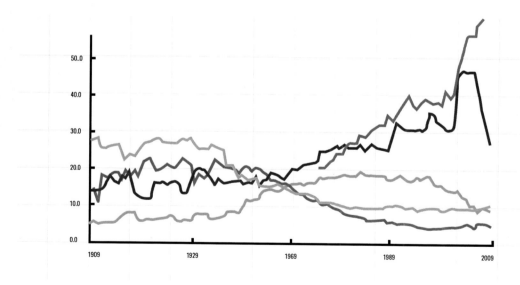

X: Year | **Y:** LB Per Capita Per Year

— Butter — Lard — Mararine — Shortening — Oils

Source: Dr. Stephan Guyenet. The American Diet. 2012.

KETO DIET RISKS – HOW YOU CAN AVOID THEM

For those who are unfamiliar with the keto diet, it's relatively simple. The keto diet is basically a low carb, high fat diet which consists of healthy fats, moderate amounts of protein and a very strict limit on carbohydrates.

What is becoming more prominent recently as the lifestyle has become more mainstream makes me frustrated.

NUTRITION

Specifically, when micronutrition gets thrown out in favour of the low carb, high fat macros.

It basically looks like this. When someone starts a ketogenic lifestyle, the hardest part is cutting out the sugar in your diet. Sometimes, people do both sugar and carbohydrates in one go. Kudos to those people! Sugar is extremely addictive, and carbohydrates have been deemed necessary for energy ever since the low-fat brigade made their way to the top.

However, what begins to happen is this. That person begins to eat an incredibly high amount of processed foods, just because the macronutrients fit the ratios required. They discard nutritious foods just because the macro nutrition of vegetables doesn't fit the strict food rules that the keto diet implies.

It often gets to the point where instead of eating living plants, natural foods, and drinking water, they substitute everything they can with a low carb alternative that is either filled with preservatives, artificially sweetened with aspartame, or has lived in a can for the past four years.

How many carbs does a cigarette have? – Is it good for your health? NO.

Hypothetically, eating a diet solely consisting of cheese will help you lose weight. This might work for the first weight loss goal because you've effectively cut out all the insulin-raising foods that prevented you from losing weight in the first place. But if you want to look after your health, then you really need to learn to understand what you're actually eating, regardless of the carbohydrate and fat content.

The biggest keto diet risks come from ignoring your body and nutrition.

So many people are deficient in many of the vital micronutrients because all they eat is salami and artificial cheese sticks. Some of these include magnesium, zinc and vitamins A, B, C and D.

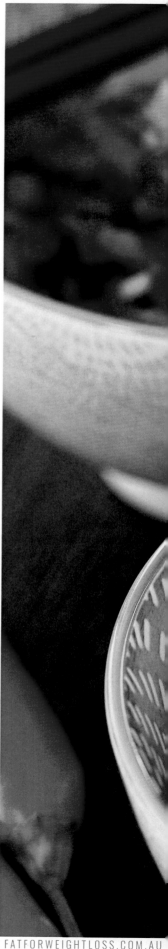

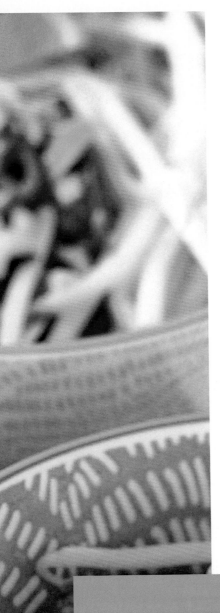

You need to teach your body to re-learn what it actually needs, instead of switching from coke to diet coke, or bakery goods to an entire box of low carb sugar-free cookies. The physical food needs to change, but so does your mindset about eating food.

My aim throughout this website is to teach you which items/mindsets are important to change for lifelong success.

Don't jump off a cliff with everyone else. Make sure you are eating healthy fats, nutritious sources of protein and a low carbohydrate content. Don't blindly follow everything you read.

Most of all, where ever possible, make those food choices organic, ethically sourced or free from known carcinogens listed here.

I'M NOT LOSING WEIGHT. WHAT AM I DOING WRONG?

Many people decide to start a ketogenic lifestyle initially to lose weight. Remember, you're not doing anything wrong if you are not losing weight. At first, the weight seems to slide off due to the water loss by restricting carbohydrates, however, after a while you might not be seeing the results that you loved during the start of the lifestyle.

This is because by eating less sugar and carbohydrates, you begin to increase your insulin sensitivity, which enables your body to build muscle.

To avoid disappointment, make sure you take body measurements when the number on the scales isn't going down. Progress pictures can give a visual representation of where you are in your ketogenic journey, but it is useful to track your waist, butt, and arm measurements.

During plateaus, you will still be shedding inches, but the scale might not necessarily move as quickly. Just keep going for the sake of whom you want to become. Just remember, Keep Calm and Keto On!

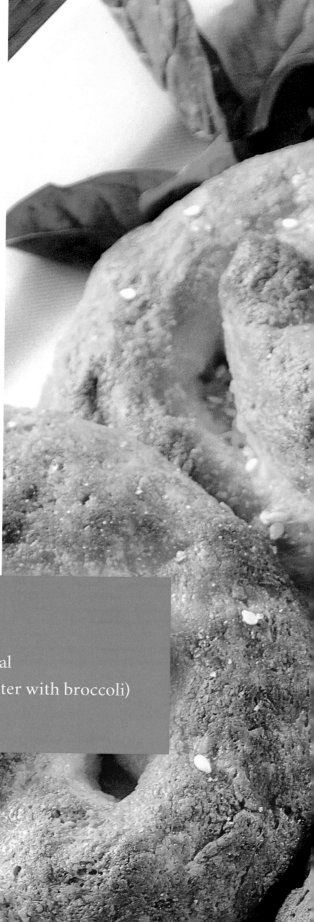

BUT THE LABEL SAYS SUGAR-FREE!

Just because the food wrapper says it is sugar-free, it does not mean it has no carbs. Or just because it is beef jerky, it does not mean it has no sugar. I've fallen into this trap a few times, turning around the packet to realize that its full of sugar!

Honestly, there are not that many keto friendly foods on the shelves at the supermarket. Keep to the outer edges of the supermarket and avoid the isles where all the packaged food is positioned. Every time you go, write down new foods that are keto friendly. In a couple of months, you will have a full list of foods that you can eat at your store.

I LIKE "INSERT FAVOURITE JUNK FOOD". CAN I EAT LOW CARB REPLACEMENTS?

One of the first things I did, when switching to keto is finding replacements for my favorite junk foods. Pizza, chips, pastries, cookies, fast foods. The problem I have with low carb replacements is I would still overeat and not hit my macros.

I had to go back, change my lifestyle, and stick to veggies, meats, and healthy fats. Once I thought of it as a lifestyle change and not a diet, it became much easier for me.

To make it really easy:

- Eat a palm-sized piece of protein with every meal
- Use vegetables as fat delivery systems (think butter with broccoli)
- Limit carbs.

Once you have been in Ketosis for a while (a few months), you can enter Ketosis again very easily, generally within two days.

However, if you are just starting out, make sure you stick with it for a while to see the real benefits before falling off the bandwagon. The results will speak for themselves!

JUST ONE WON'T HURT, RIGHT?

Just because the food wrapper says it is sugar-free, it does Let's admit it; most people have cheat days in their diet. You are not going to die if you eat a donut. For me, it becomes a slippery slope, where a cheat day becomes a cheat week.

Practice self-control. The trick that I learned is not to trust my first instinct. If you are in a cafeteria and you tell yourself that you want a donut, tell yourself that your first instinct is incorrect when it comes to food.

Some people have pictures on their phone to remind them where they were on the journey a couple of months ago to help them not cheat.

However, if you must cheat every now and again, don't think that you've ruined everything, just make sure you get back on track. Meal plans and meal preparation are key processes that make your life easier as you begin a ketogenic lifestyle.

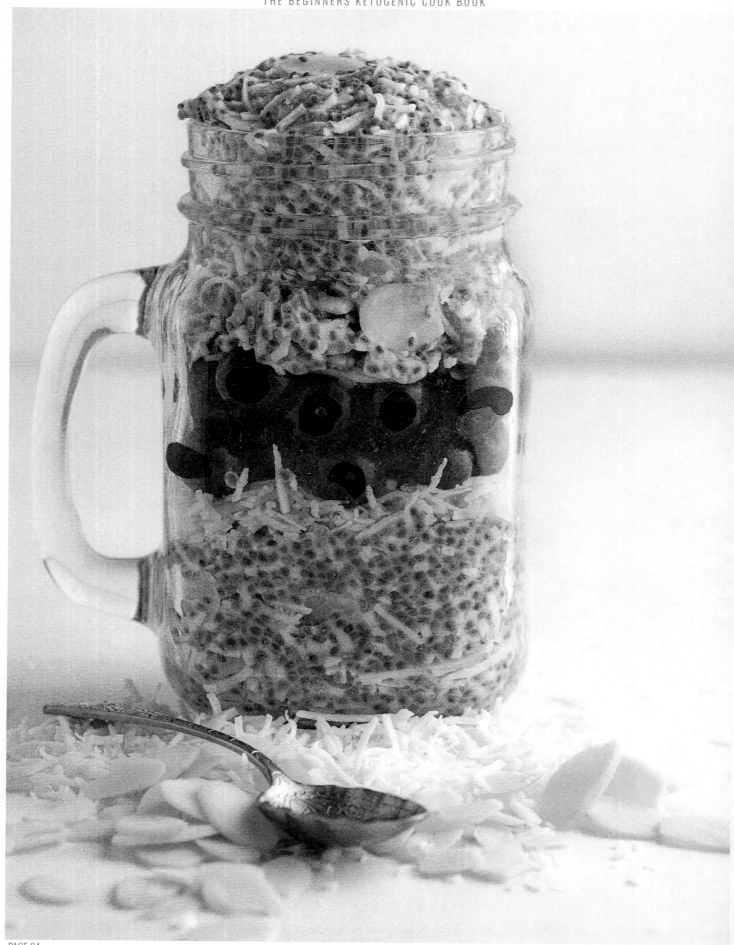

OATMEAL

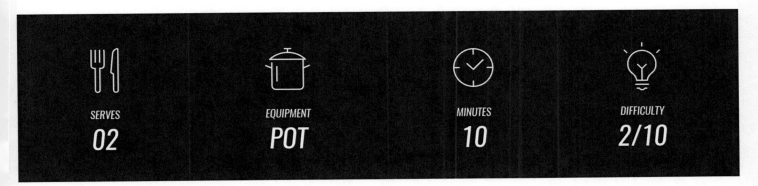

SERVES	EQUIPMENT	MINUTES	DIFFICULTY
02	POT	10	2/10

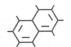

NUTRITIONAL INFORMATION PER SERVING:

480 CALORIES | 10 G CARBS | 38 G FAT | 12 G PROTEIN

INGREDIENTS

- **1/4 cup** chia seeds
- **1/4 cup** shredded coconut
- **1/3 cup** flaked coconut or more shredded coconut
- **1/3 cup** flaked almonds

- **1 tsp** vanilla extract
- **1/2 cup** coconut milk
- **1 cup** water
- **5-10 drops** stevia extract

PROCEDURE

(Optional bonus points - In a frying pan brown the Flaked Coconut and Flaked Almonds for about 2 mins)

Add all ingredients to a pot on the stove on medium

Cook for 7-10 mins on medium-high stirring every 30 seconds.

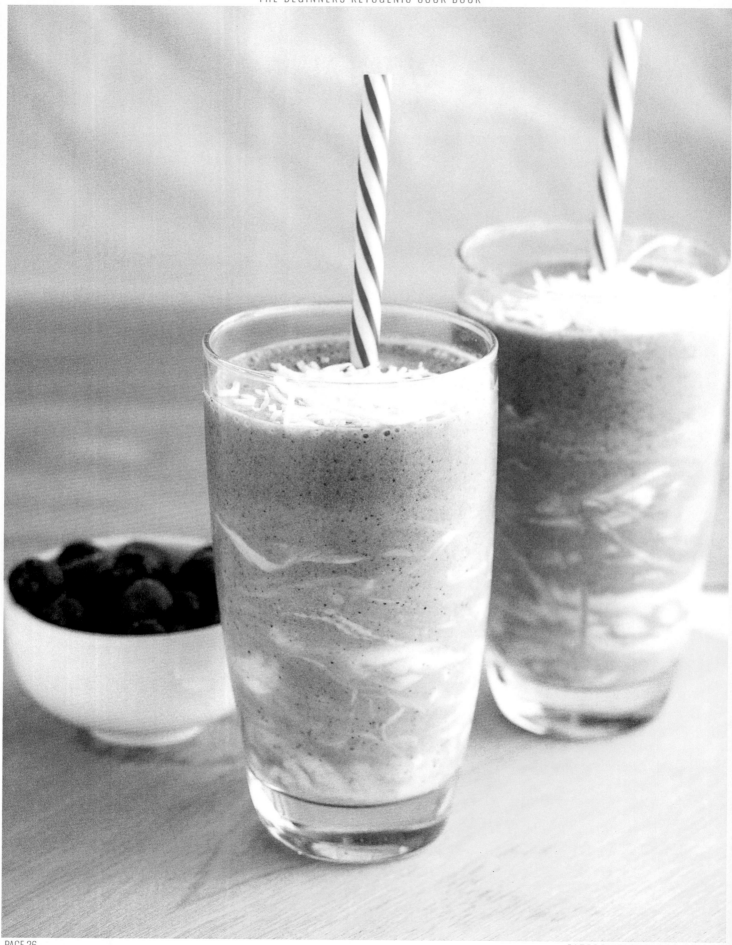

BLUEBERRY GALAXY KETO SMOOTHIE

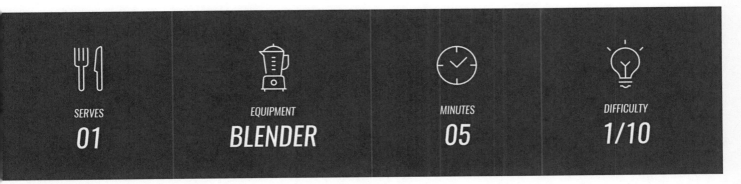

SERVES	EQUIPMENT	MINUTES	DIFFICULTY
01	**BLENDER**	**05**	**1/10**

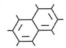

NUTRITIONAL INFORMATION PER SERVING:

282 CALORIES | **05 G CARBS** | **18.9 G FAT** | **21 G PROTEIN**

INGREDIENTS

- **1 cup** coconut milk
- **1/4 cup** blueberries
- **1 tsp** vanilla extract

- **1 tsp** MCT oil
- **1 scoop** protein powder
  (optional)

PROCEDURE

Put all the ingredients into a mixer, and blend until smooth.

If you like the swirl, I added a tablespoon of some full fat yogurt after the smoothie was in the cup, and swirled it around, touching the sides.

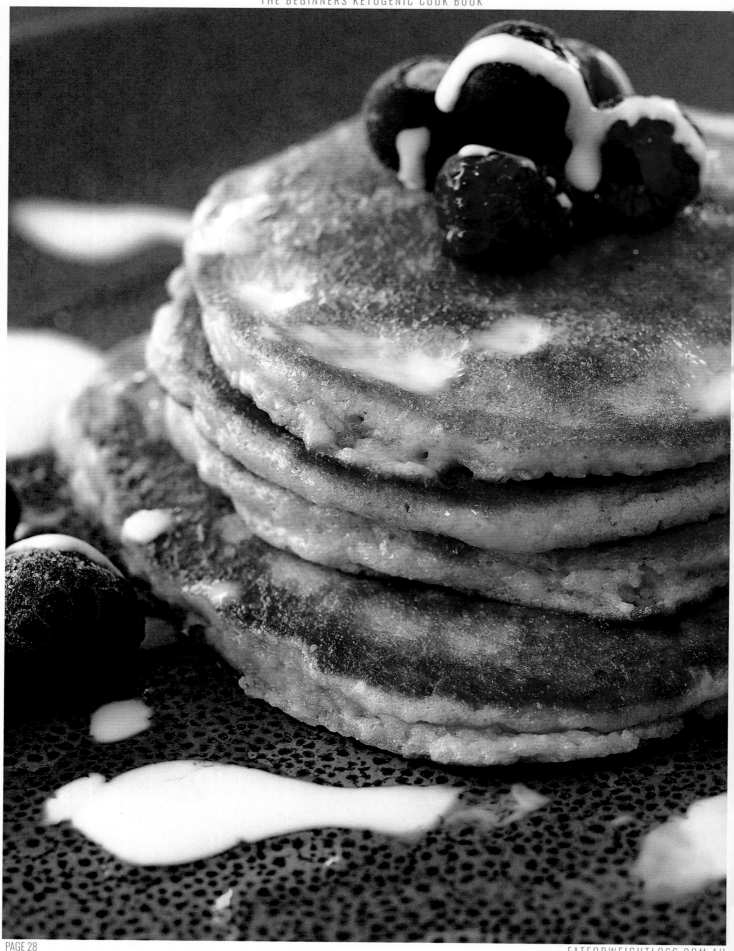

PANCAKES

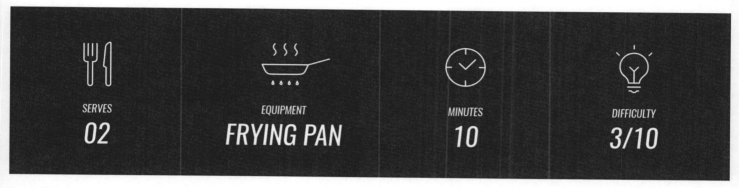

SERVES	EQUIPMENT	MINUTES	DIFFICULTY
02	FRYING PAN	10	3/10

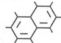

NUTRITIONAL INFORMATION:

363 CALORIES | 04 G CARBS | 32 G FAT | 12 G PROTEIN

INGREDIENTS

- **2** Eggs
- **1/2 cup** almond flour
- **2 tbsp** coconut oil (*melted*)
- **1 tsp** vanilla extract

- **2 tbsp** erythritol
- **1/4 tsp** baking soda
- **1/2 tsp** cream of tartar

PROCEDURE

Beat the eggs with an electric mixer, add the cream of tatar and continue mixing.

Slowly, Add the almond flour into the mix. Add the melted coconut oil, vanilla extract, baking soda and erythritol.

If necessary, add 1 Tbsp. water to the mix to find desired consistency.

Heat up a frying pan and pour mixture slowly into desired shape.

Serve with berries, cream and enjoy!

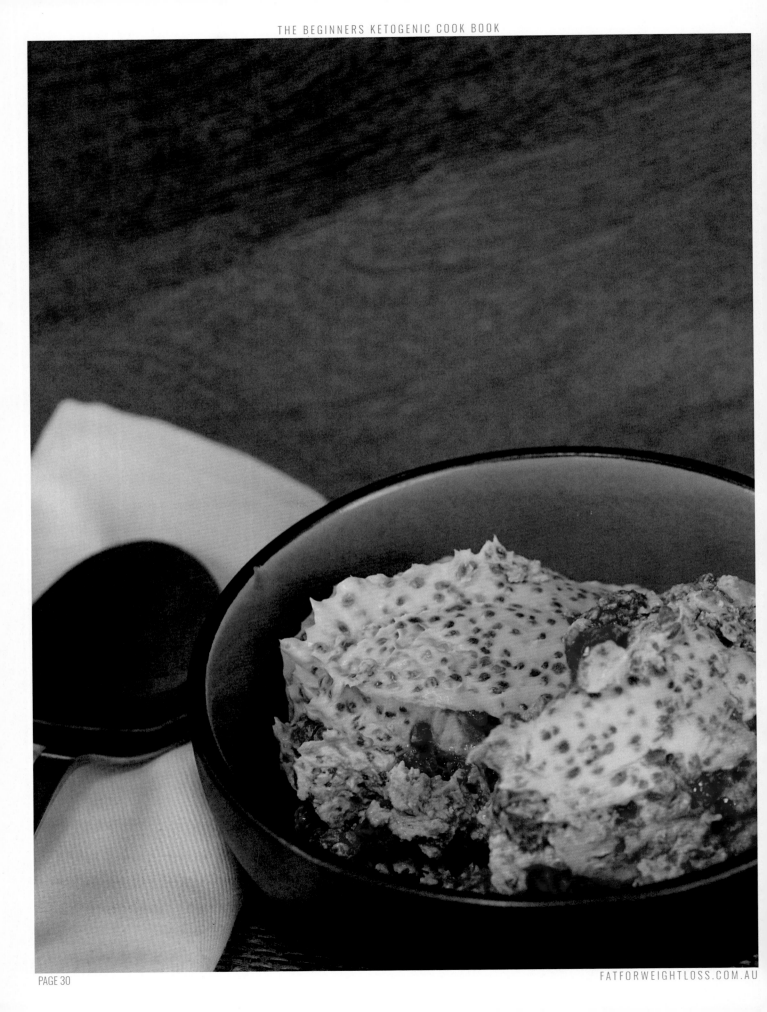

RASPBERRY COCONUT CHIA SEED PUDDING

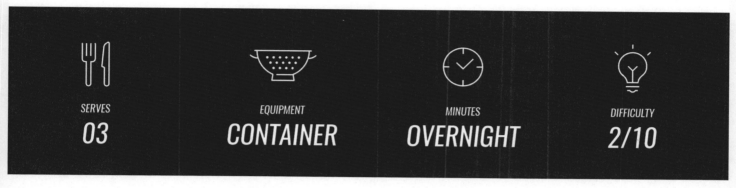

SERVES
03

EQUIPMENT
CONTAINER

MINUTES
OVERNIGHT

DIFFICULTY
2/10

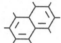

NUTRITIONAL INFORMATION PER SERVING:

368 CALORIES | 02 G CARBS | 33 G FAT | 03 G PROTEIN

INGREDIENTS

- **2 cups** coconut cream (*13.5 oz / 400ml*)
- **3 tbsp** chia seeds
- **1 tsp** vanilla extract
- **1/4 cup** frozen berries (*raspberries*)

PROCEDURE

Get a container and place the coconut cream inside.

Add the chia seeds and mix around with a spoon.

Add the vanilla extract and the frozen berries.

Place in the fridge overnight. The chia seeds should expand and become soft, squishy and delicious.

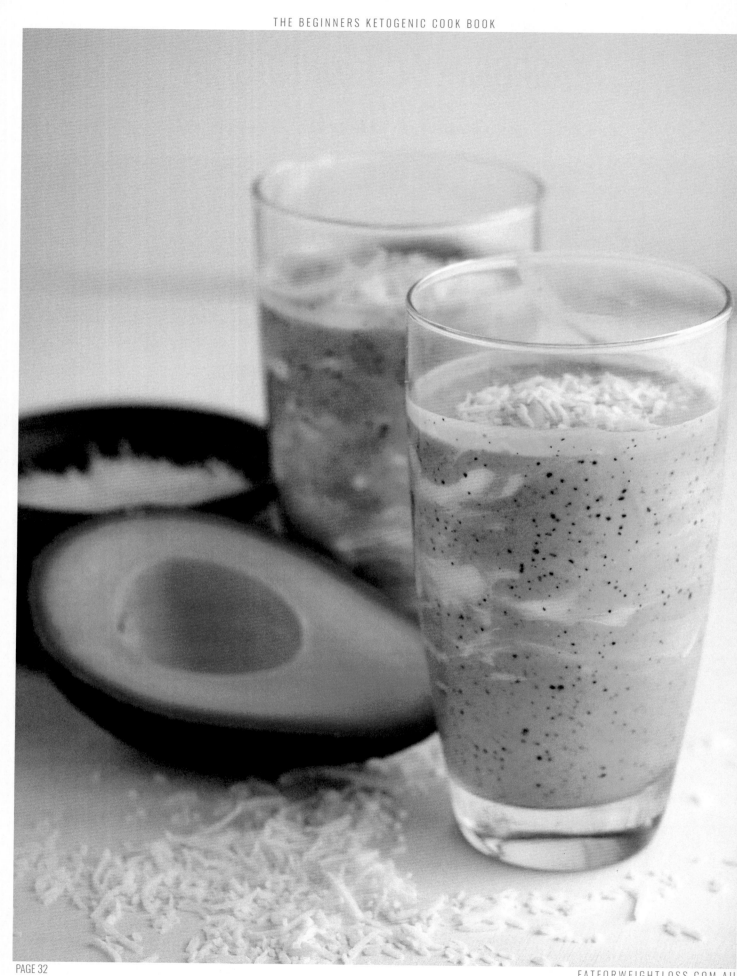

AVOCADO SMOOTHIE

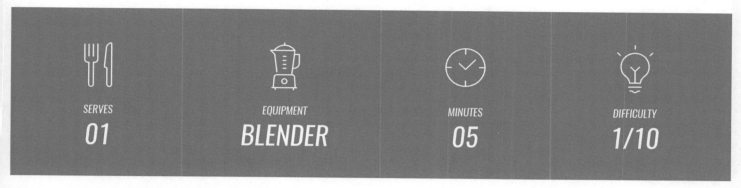

SERVES
01

EQUIPMENT
BLENDER

MINUTES
05

DIFFICULTY
1/10

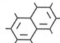

NUTRITIONAL INFORMATION PER SERVING:

244 CALORIES | **06 G CARBS** | **20 G FAT** | **03 G PROTEIN**

INGREDIENTS

- **1 cup** coconut milk
- **1/2** whole avocado
- **1 cup** spinach

- **1/4 cup** blueberries
- **1 tsp** vanilla extract
- **1 tsp** MCT oil

PROCEDURE

Put all the ingredients into a mixer, and blend until smooth.

If you like the swirl, I added a tablespoon of some full fat yogurt after the smoothie was in the cup, and swirled it around, touching the sides.

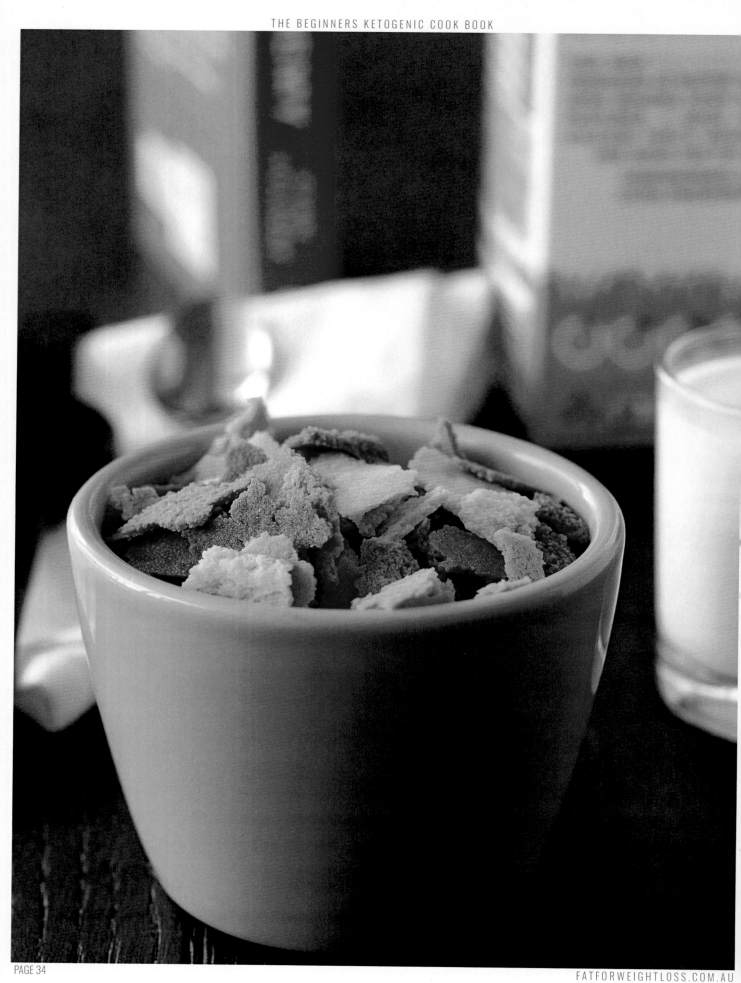

"CORN" FLAKES

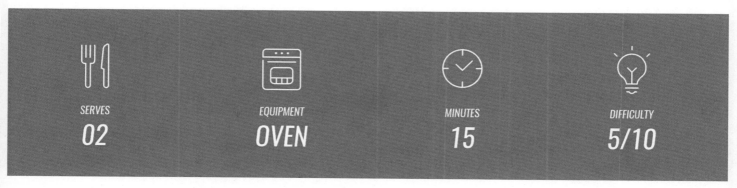

SERVES
02

EQUIPMENT
OVEN

MINUTES
15

DIFFICULTY
5/10

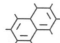

NUTRITIONAL INFORMATION PER SERVING:

328 CALORIES | **06 G CARBS** | **28 G FAT** | **12 G PROTEIN**

INGREDIENTS

- **1 cup** almond meal
- **1 tbsp** erythritol
- **1/2 tsp** salt
- **1 tsp** vanilla extract
- **3/4 cups** water

PROCEDURE

Preheat oven to 320 F (*160 C*) degrees. Line a baking tray with baking paper (*Parchment paper*) and grease lightly with butter.

Whisk together almond flour, erythritol and salt. Add vanilla extract and water.

Pour mixture onto prepared pan and spread out evenly. You want a nice thin layer.

Bake for 10-15 minutes, keeping a close eye on it, until the mixture has dried out and cracked.

Remove from oven, let it cool, then use your hands to tear and crack the dough into small flakes.

Return to oven and let bake on the center rack for about 10 minutes or until pieces are toasted, crisp, and golden.

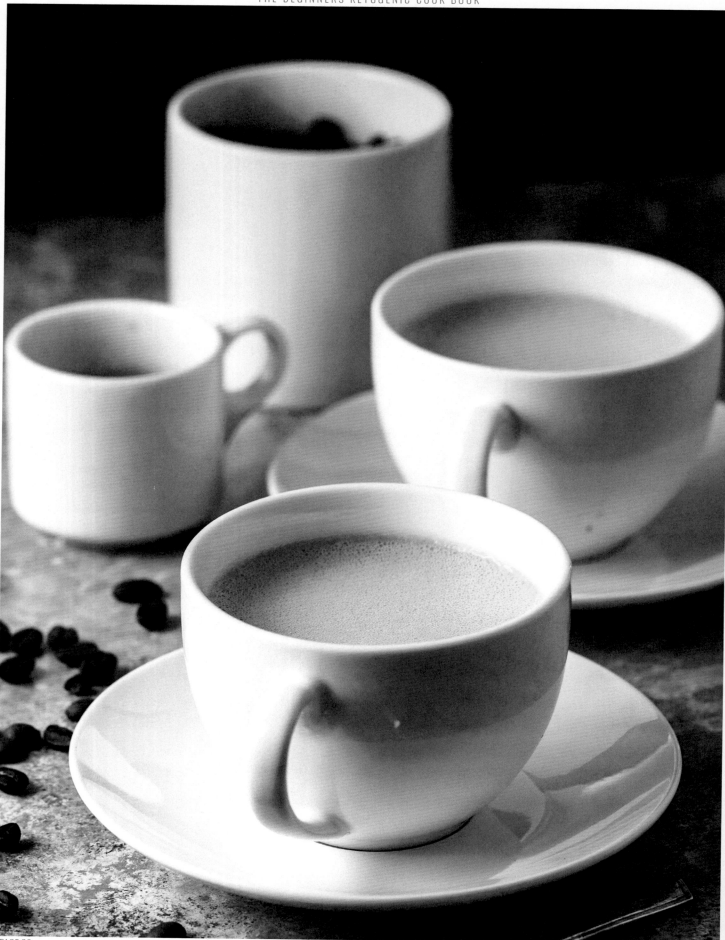

BEGINNERS BUTTER COFFEE

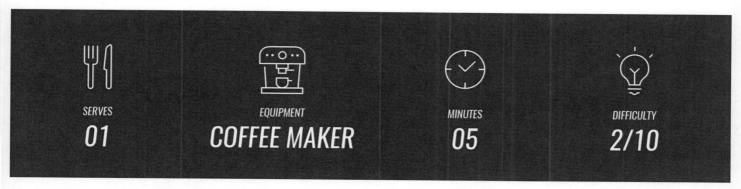

SERVES
01

EQUIPMENT
COFFEE MAKER

MINUTES
05

DIFFICULTY
2/10

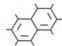

NUTRITIONAL INFORMATION:

143 CALORIES | **0 G CARBS** | **16 G FAT** | **0 G PROTEIN**

INGREDIENTS

- **1 cup** black coffee
- **1 Tbsp** cream
- **1 tsp** MCT oil *(Or Coconut Oil)*

PROCEDURE

Make the black coffee however you like

Add the cream and the black coffee into a blender.

(Please make sure your blender can blend hot water before trying).

Add 1 teaspoon of MCT Oil to the mix and blend for 30 seconds.

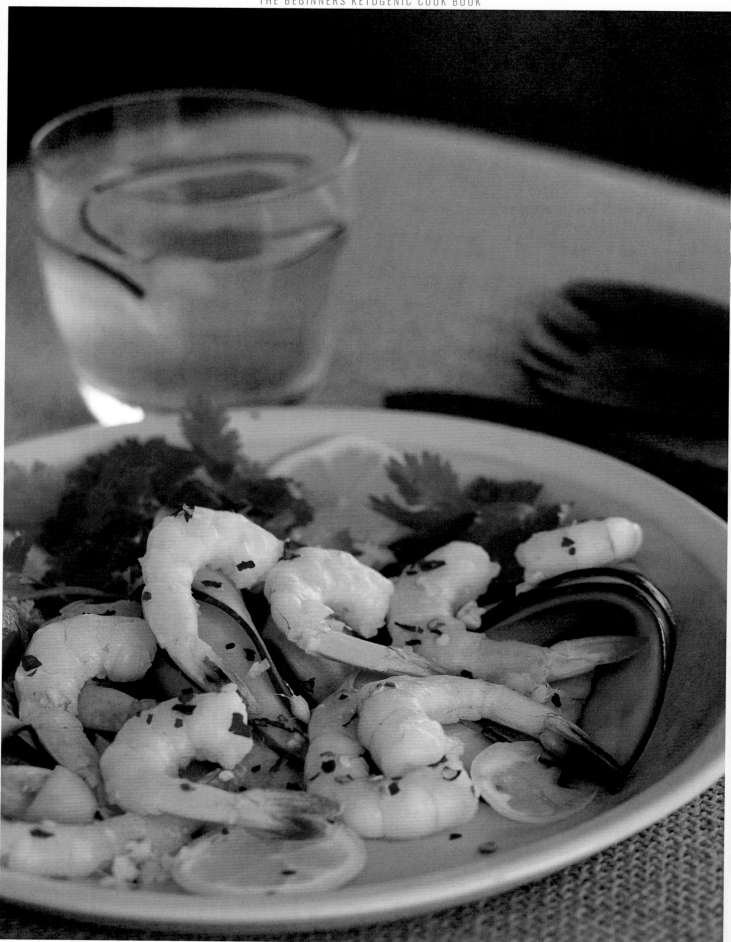

HOT SPICY PRAWNS WITH COOL CUCUMBER SALAD

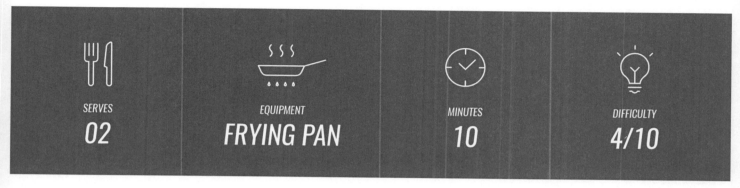

SERVES
02

EQUIPMENT
FRYING PAN

MINUTES
10

DIFFICULTY
4/10

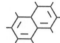

NUTRITIONAL INFORMATION:

602 CALORIES | **03 G CARBS** | **47 G FAT** | **37 G PROTEIN**

INGREDIENTS

- **12 oz** fresh prawns (*peeled 350g*)
- **2** cucumbers (*200g / 7oz*)
- **1.5 oz** butter (*50g*)
- **3 tbsp** olive oil
- **1 tbsp** sesame seed oil

- **1 tsp** fresh ginger
- **2 tbsp** fresh lemon juice
- **1** red chili (or chili flakes)
- **4** garlic cloves
- salt and pepper to taste

PROCEDURE

Heat the butter and olive oil in a medium frying pan, when medium hot add the ginger, chili and garlic.

When you begin to smell the flavors, add the prawns a cook for 2 mins until slightly pink. Remove from pan and let cool slightly.

Peel the entire cucumber with a peeler into long strips.

Cover with sesame seed oil and lemon.

Add the prawns onto the bed of cucumber, add salt and pepper to taste. Serve with cucumber sparkling water.

ASIAN STEAMED SESAME CHICKEN

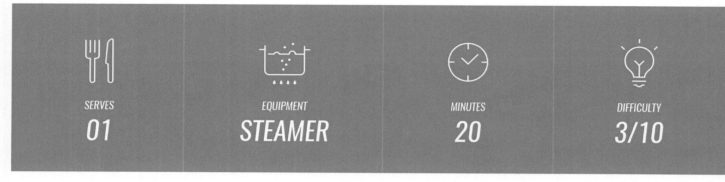

SERVES
01

EQUIPMENT
STEAMER

MINUTES
20

DIFFICULTY
3/10

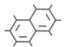

NUTRITIONAL INFORMATION:

625 CALORIES | **10 G CARBS** | **38 G FAT** | **55 G PROTEIN**

INGREDIENTS

- **1** chicken breast
- **1** bunch bok choy
- **1** handful shallots
- **1 tsp** minced ginger
- **2 tbsp** sesame seed oil

PROCEDURE

Bring a large pot of water to boil with the steamer on top. Slice the chicken breast from side to side *(as if you where to butterfly)* and place the chicken in the steamer for 10 mins each side.

As the timer hits 15 mins, add the bok choy into the steamer and cook for 5 mins.

Whilst the ingredients are cooking, chop the shallots and ginger and add them to a bowl. Add the sesame seed oil and mix together to form a sauce.

Place the chicken on a plate and cover with the sauce.

Enjoy!

OVEN BAKED CHICKEN WINGS WITH LIME COCONUT SAUCE

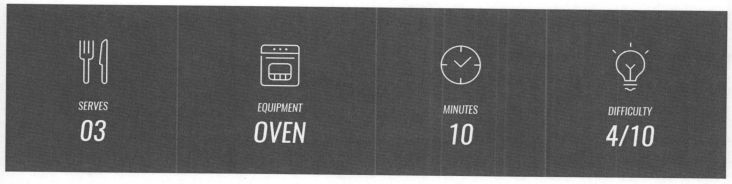

SERVES	EQUIPMENT	MINUTES	DIFFICULTY
03	**OVEN**	**10**	**4/10**

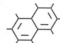

NUTRITIONAL INFORMATION:

735 CALORIES | **03 G CARBS** | **61 G FAT** | **38 G PROTEIN**

INGREDIENTS

WINGS
- **17.5 oz** chicken wings (500g)
- **3.5 oz** butter melted (100 g)
- **1 tbsp** paprika
- **1/4 tbsp** cayenne pepper

SAUCE
- **1/2 cup** coconut cream
- **1/2** avocado
- **1/2** lime
- **1 tbsp** sesame seed oil
- **1/4 tsp** lime skin
- **1 tsp** salt
- **1 tsp** pepper

PROCEDURE

Place chicken wings on a baking tray and bake in the oven at 375 F (*180 C*) for 45 mins or until golden brown.

Whilst the chicken wings are in the oven, Add all of the sauce ingredients into a blender (*I used a Nutribullet).* I just cut a lime in half and added the whole thing, skin, pulp and all. It makes for a wonderfully tangy taste. Blend until completely smooth.

Melt the butter and add the paprika and cayenne pepper. Mix this in a bowl large enough to fit all the chicken wings in once they are cooked.

Once the wings are cooked and crispy on the outside, place them in the same bowl with the butter and seasonings, and coat, swish and baste them liberally in the delicious fatty goodness. Plate them and serve with the sauce.

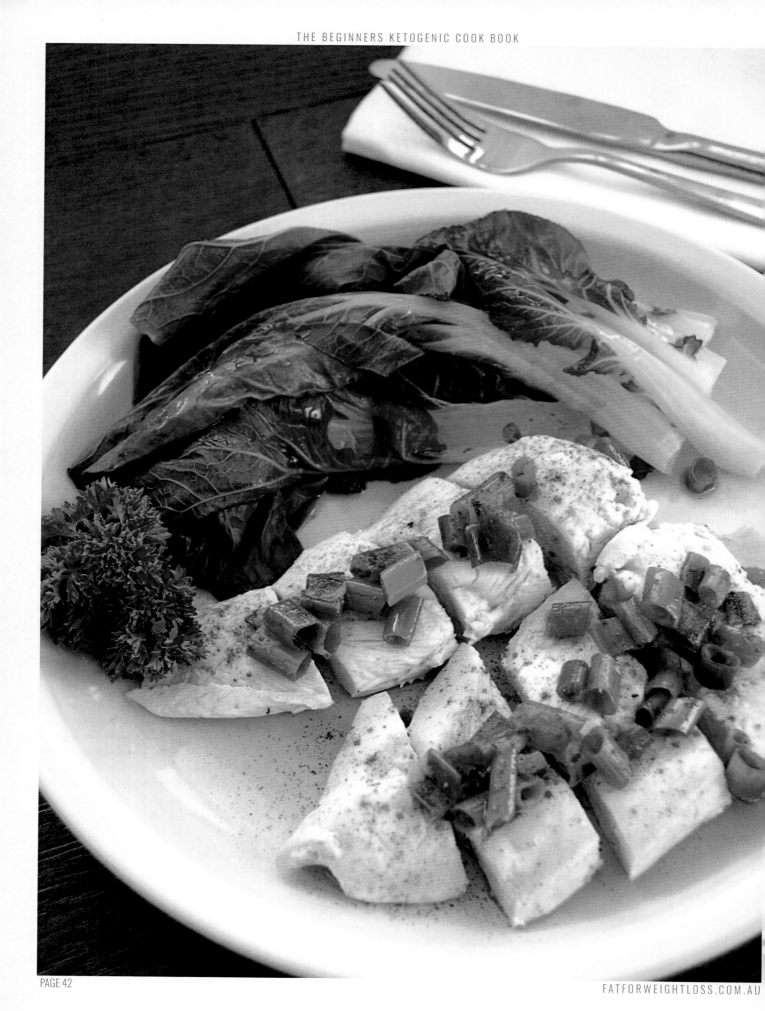

CREAMY CHICKEN AVOCADO SALAD WITH SESAME SAUCE

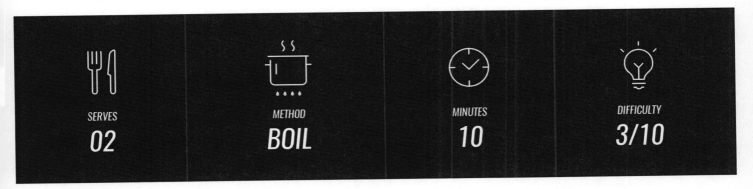

SERVES	METHOD	MINUTES	DIFFICULTY
02	BOIL	10	3/10

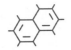

NUTRITIONAL INFORMATION:

425 CALORIES | **02 G CARBS** | **23 G FAT** | **32 G PROTEIN**

INGREDIENTS

- **1** chicken breast
- **3** cherry tomatoes
- **1/2** avocado
- **1 tbsp** red onion

- **2 tbsp** sesame seed oil
- **1** handful lettuce
- **2 tbsp** mayonnaise
- **1 tsp** paprika optional

PROCEDURE

Place the chicken breast on a baking tray and cook at 180° C *(375° F)* for 20 mins *(optionally add paprika to the top of the chicken breast at this point).*

Cut up the salad ingredients to your liking, place on a plate *(usually I use the lettuce as a bed to place all the other ingredients on).*

Cut the chicken into pieces and place onto salad. Mix the mayonnaise with the sesame seed oil and use as a dressing.

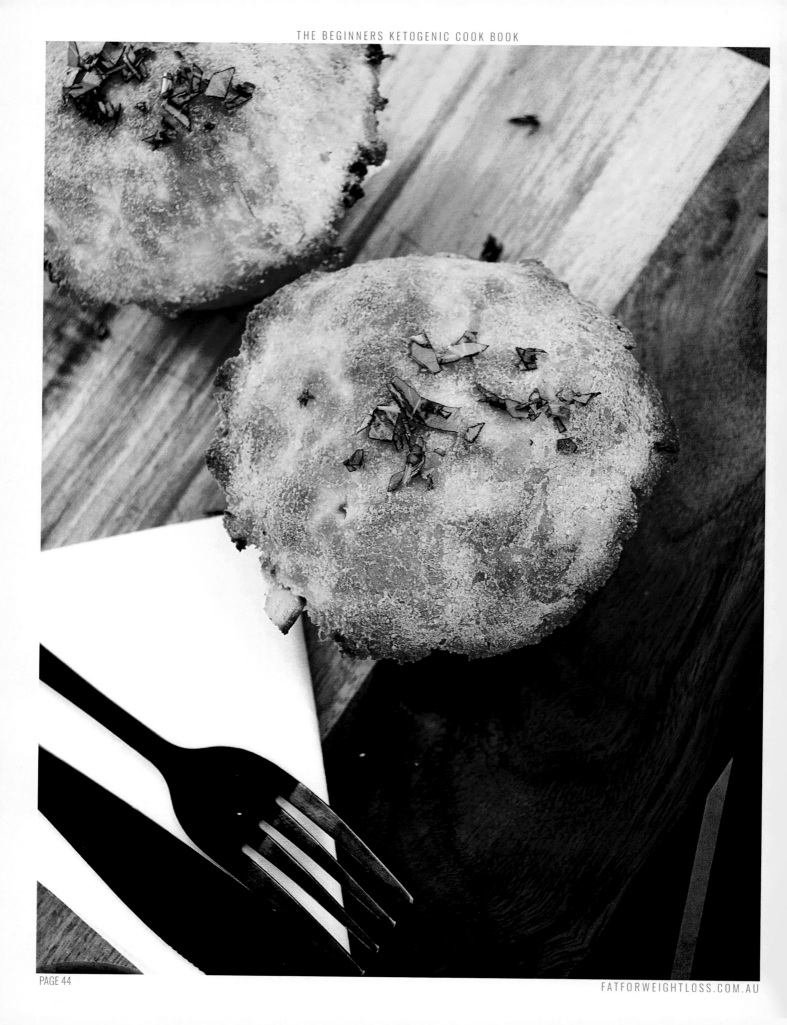

MEAT PIE

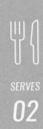

SERVES
02

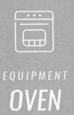

EQUIPMENT
OVEN

MINUTES
30

DIFFICULTY
7/10

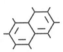

NUTRITIONAL INFORMATION:

970 CALORIES | 10 G CARBS | 79 G FAT | 51 G PROTEIN

INGREDIENTS

PIE CRUST

- **1/2 cup** coconut flour
- **1/4** water
- **2 oz** butter (chilled / 60g)

PIE TOP

- **1/2 cup** mozzarella cheese
- **1 tbsp** coconut flour
- **1 egg**

PIE MINCE

- **7 oz** mince *(200g)*
- **2 tbsp** olive oil
- **1/2** carrot
- **1/2** onion
- **1** stock cube
- **6.5 fl/oz** water *(200 ml)*
- **1 tsp** xanthan gum
- **1 tbsp** tomato sauce sugar free
- **1 tsp** gelatin *(optional thickener)*

PROCEDURE

Add crust ingredients into bowl and mix with a fork. The butter will be hard to press, but stick with it!

Place the ingredients into a small pie pan and press out the bottom and edges. I used a measuring cup to do all the hard work for me. Place in the fridge while you get the filling ready.

In a pan, add the onion first with the olive oil.

Add the meat and remaining vegetables until the mince is cooked. Place the remaining ingredients into the pan and let it simmer for 5 mins. The liquid should thicken nicely.

Remove the pie crust from the fridge and fill with the meat.

Melt the mozzarella cheese in the microwave for 60 secs, add the coconut flour and egg until it resembles dough. Roll out into round pie crust toppings.

Place in the oven at 180 C *(360 F)* for 15-20 mins *(until top is brown)*.

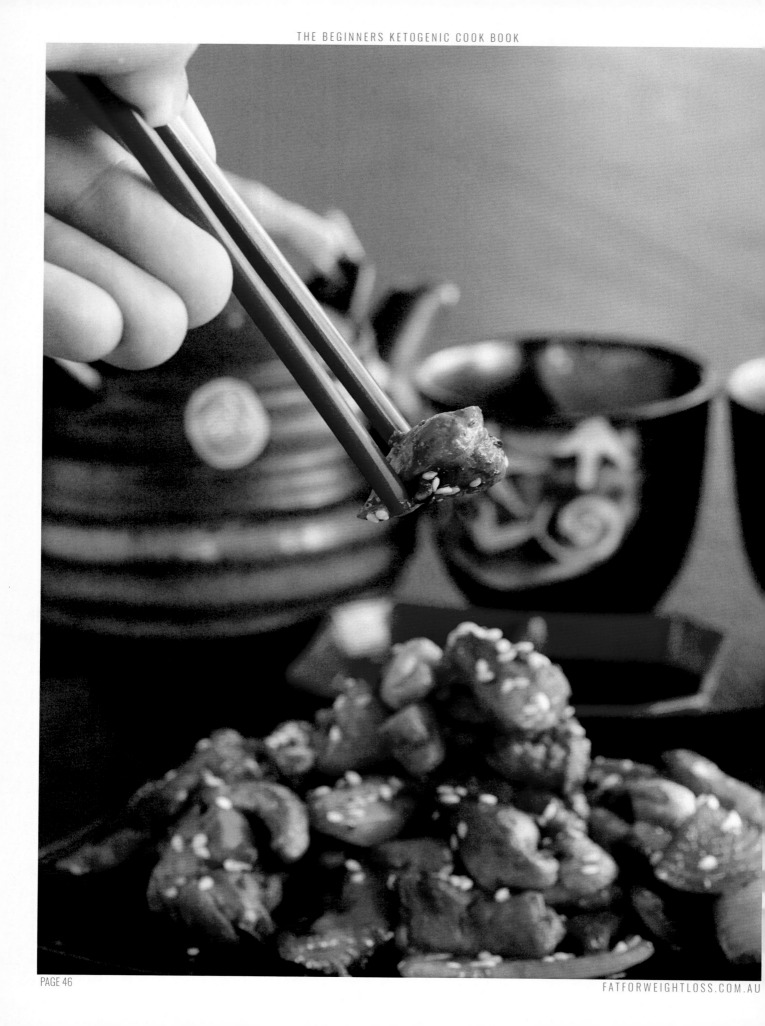

CHILI CASHEW CHICKEN

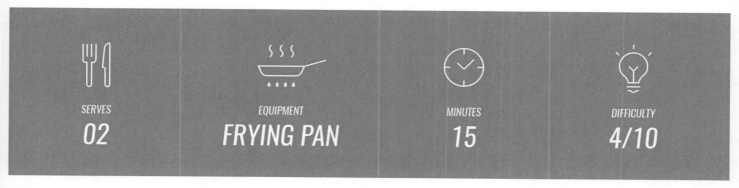

SERVES
02

EQUIPMENT
FRYING PAN

MINUTES
15

DIFFICULTY
4/10

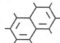

NUTRITIONAL INFORMATION:

562 CALORIES | 07 G CARBS | 48 G FAT | 27 G PROTEIN

INGREDIENTS

- **3** chicken thighs
- **2 tbsp** coconut oil
- **1/2** capsicum (*green pepper*)
- **1/4** white onion
- **1 tbsp** shallots (*green onions*)
- **1/2 tsp** fresh ginger

- **1/4 cup** cashews
- **1 tbsp** rice wine vinegar
- **2 tbsp** soy sauce (*gluten free*)
- **2 tbsp** sesame oil
- **1 tbsp** sesame seeds
- **1 tbsp** fresh chili (*or chili flakes*)

PROCEDURE

Cut the chicken and onion into 1 inch chunks.

Cook only the chicken on high in the coconut oil for 4 - 5 mins.

Add the capsicum, onions, garlic, ginger, fresh chili. Cook on high for another 2-3 minutes.

Add the Rice wine vinegar, soy sauce and the cashews. Reduce the heat and simmer until liquid reduces.

Top with sesames seeds and enjoy!

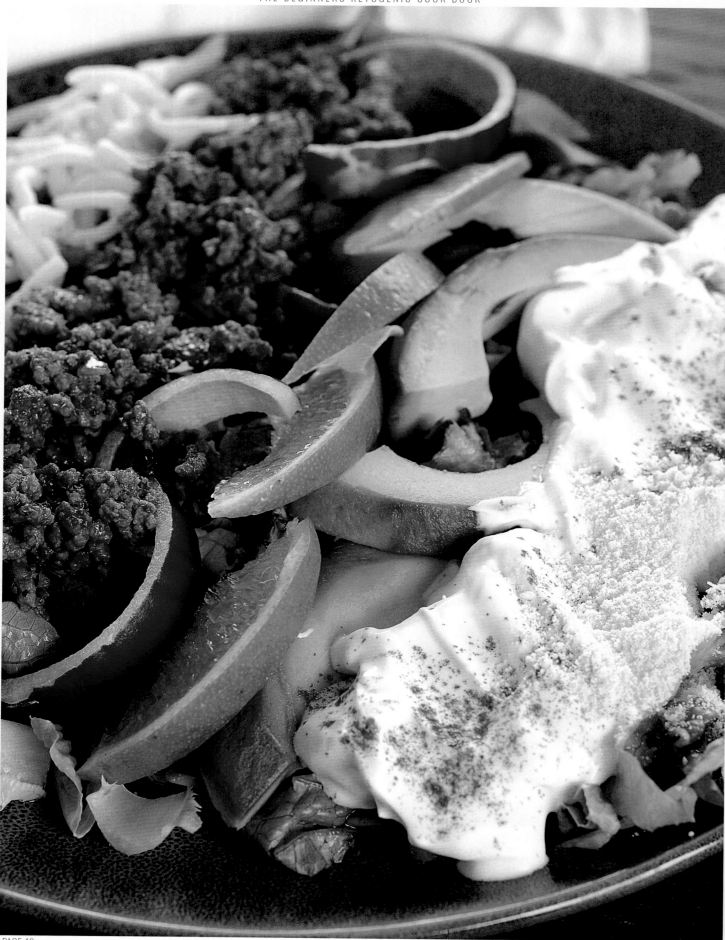

TACO SALAD

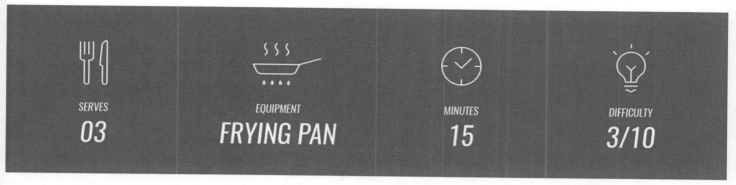

SERVES
03

EQUIPMENT
FRYING PAN

MINUTES
15

DIFFICULTY
3/10

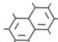

NUTRITIONAL INFORMATION:

560 CALORIES | **06 G CARBS** | **42 G FAT** | **41 G PROTEIN**

INGREDIENTS

- **1/2** cup grated cheeese
- **2 cups** chopped lettuce
- **1** avocado
- **1/2** lime
- **1/2 cup** sour cream
- **2 tbsp** red onion chopped (*optional*)
- **1 lb** beef mince (*ground beef*) (*500 g*)

SEASONING

- **1/4 tsp** garlic powder
- **1/4 tsp** dried oregano
- **1/2 tsp** paprika
- **1 ½ tsp** ground cumin
- **3/4 cup** water

PROCEDURE

Heat a frying pan and add the mince to the pan. Cook until brown. add the seasoning and 3/4 Cup of water and let it simmer for 5 mins.

Grab a plate and cover with the chopped lettuce. Cover with ingredients however you like! Enjoy.

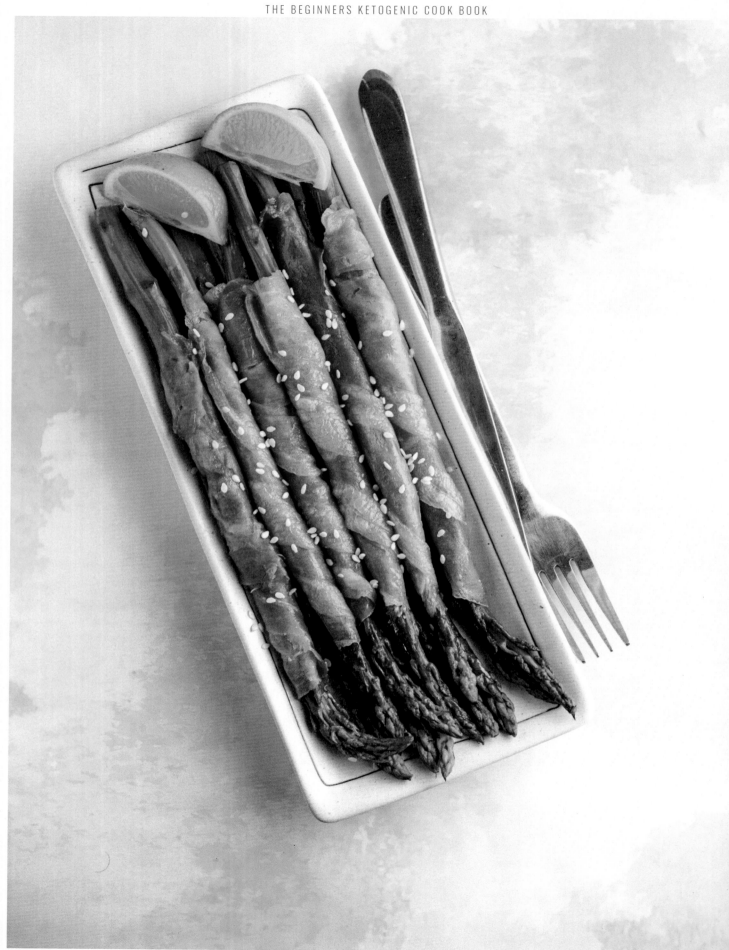

PROSCIUTTO WRAPPED ASPARAGUS

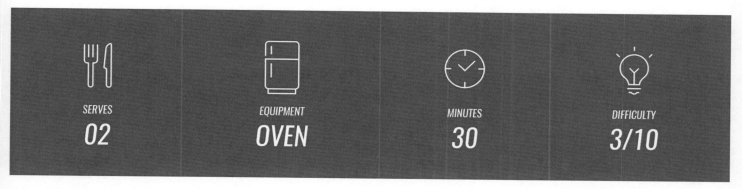

SERVES
02

EQUIPMENT
OVEN

MINUTES
30

DIFFICULTY
3/10

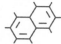

NUTRITIONAL INFORMATION:

410 CALORIES | **02 G CARBS** | **35 G FAT** | **25 G PROTEIN**

INGREDIENTS

- **16** spears asparagus (*trimmed, woody ends removed*)
- **6 slices** Prosciutto (*halved*)
- **3 tbsp** Olive Oil
- salt and pepper freshly ground

PROCEDURE

Bring a large pot of water to the boil, add the asparagus spears to the water and cook for 5 mins

Drain the water, wrap the asparagus in the prosciutto.

Place on an oven tray and baste with the olive oil. Cook for 15 mins at 350 F (180 C), turning after 7 mins.

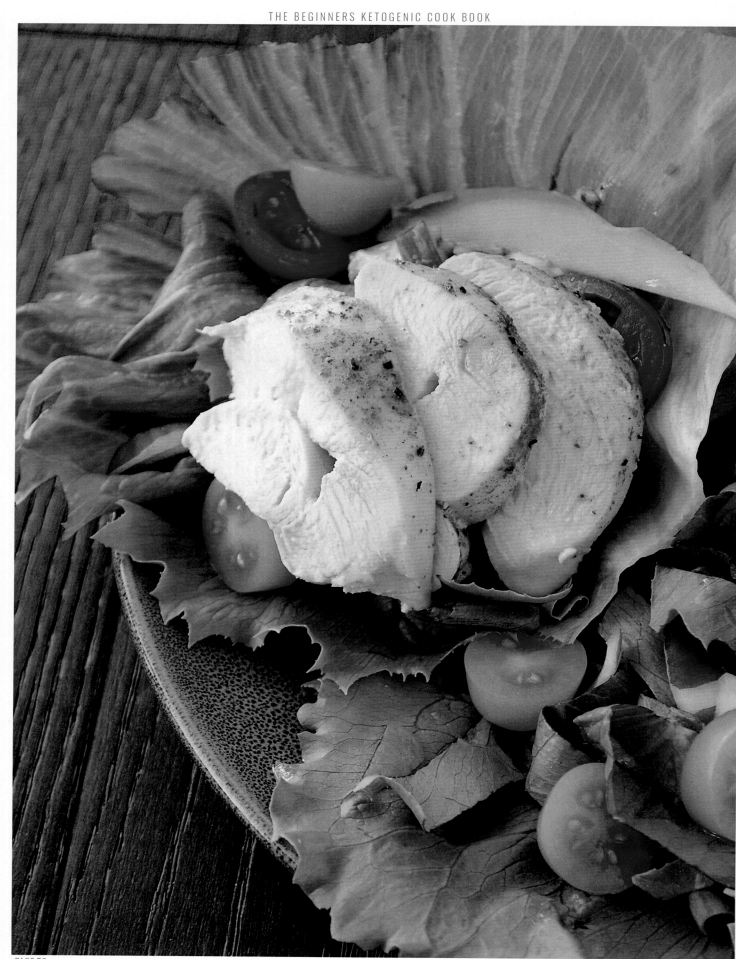

CHICKEN LETTUCE CUPS WITH CREAMY CORIANDER SAUCE

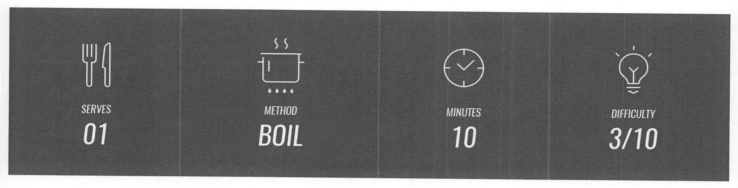

SERVES	METHOD	MINUTES	DIFFICULTY
01	BOIL	10	3/10

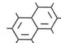

NUTRITIONAL INFORMATION:

562 CALORIES | 02 G CARBS | 48 G FAT | 27 G PROTEIN

INGREDIENTS

- **1** chicken breast
- **3** lettuce leafs
- **3** chery tomatoes
- **1 tbsp** red onion

- **3 tbsp** mayonnaise
- **1 tbsp** coriander chopped
- **1 tbsp** sesame seed oil
- salt and pepper

PROCEDURE

Place the chicken breast on a baking tray, cover with some sesame seed oil and bake at 180° C *(375° F)* for 20 mins.

Cut 3 large leaves of iceberg lettuce from the stalks to make cups. Slice up the tomatoes and red onion and fill the inside of the cup.

Slice the breast into small chunks and place inside the lettuce leafs.

Mix the mayonnaise with the coriander, add a little sesame seed oil and drip over the lettuce cups.

Cover with salt and pepper and enjoy!

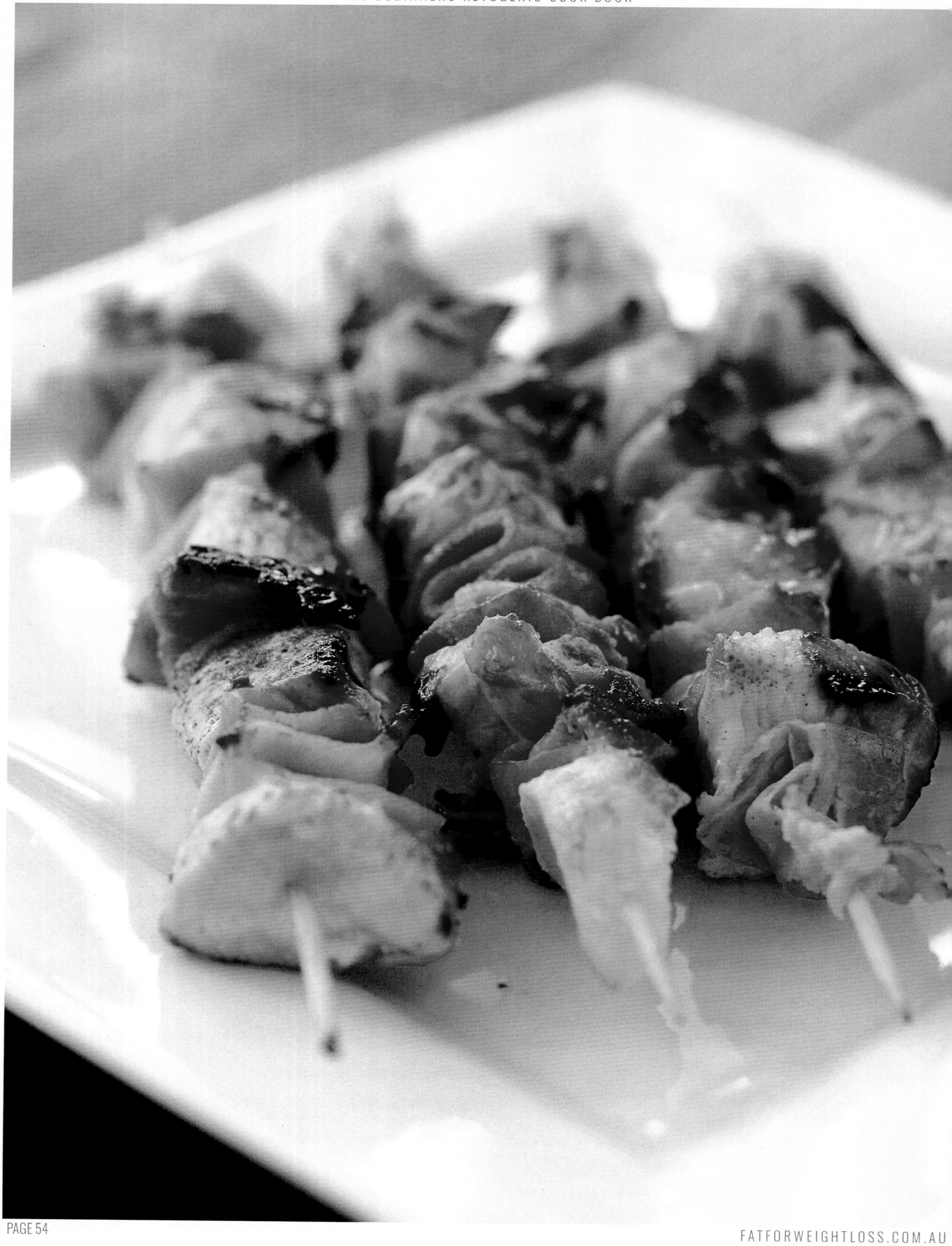

CHICKEN AND BACON SKEWERS

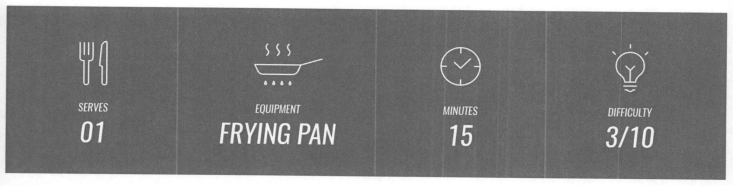

SERVES	EQUIPMENT	MINUTES	DIFFICULTY
01	FRYING PAN	15	3/10

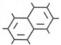

NUTRITIONAL INFORMATION:

519 CALORIES | **02 G CARBS** | **41 G FAT** | **33 G PROTEIN**

INGREDIENTS

- **3** slices bacon (100g / 3.5 oz)
- **1** chicken breast
- **2 tbsps** sesame seed oil
- **1 tsp** paprika
- bamboo skewers

PROCEDURE

Simply cut the chicken breast into chunks that are about 2cm x 2cm (roughly the size in the photo).

Cut the bacon into similar chunks and thread them onto bamboo skewers.

Sprinkle with Paprika and cook for about 5 mins each side.

Once finished, drizzle with sesame seed oil and serve!

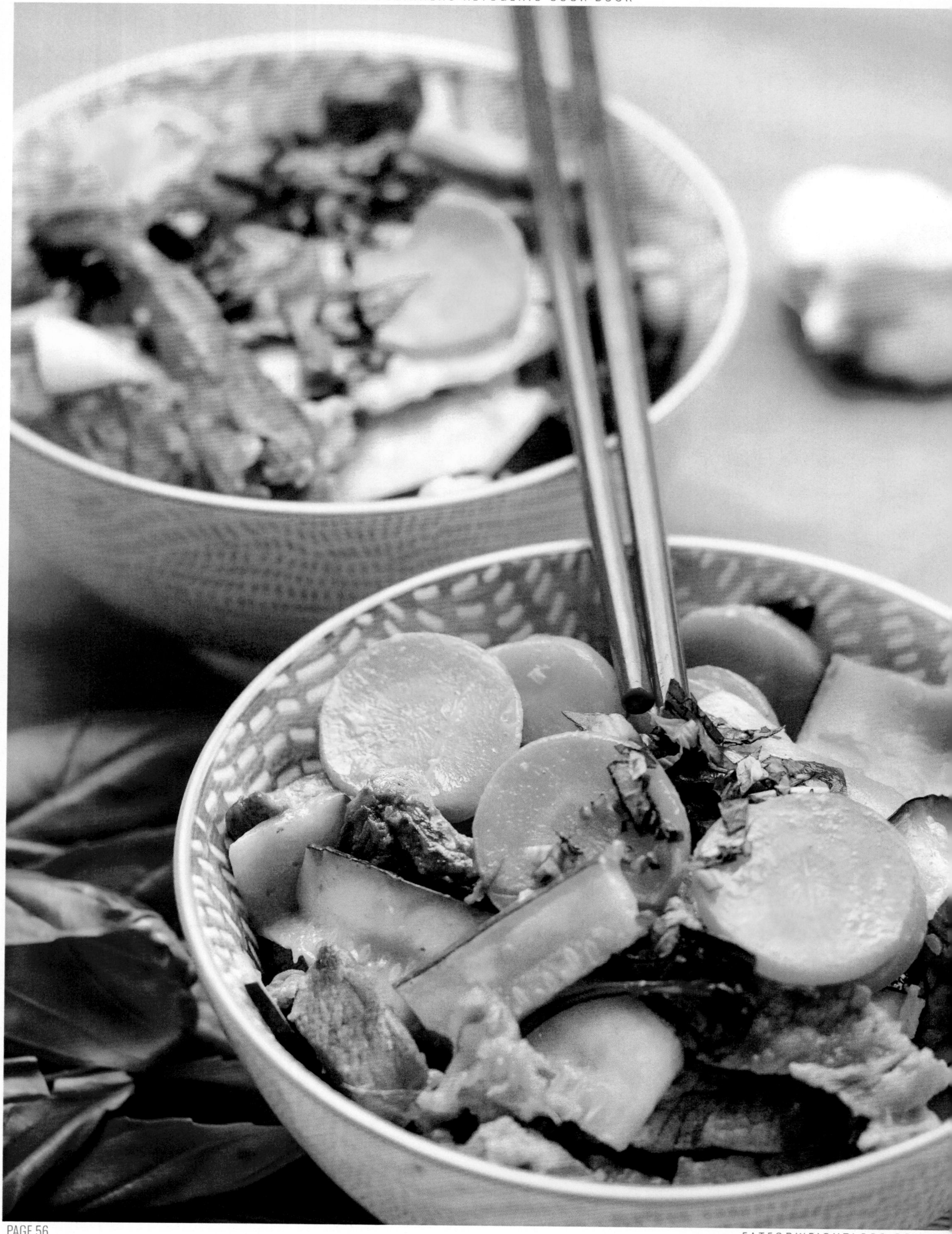

THAI BEEF STIR FRY

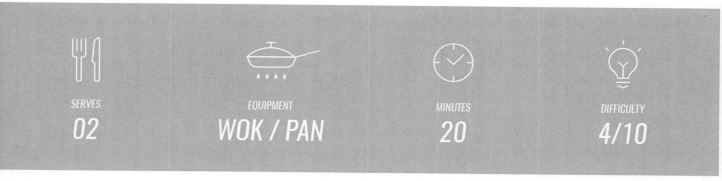

SERVES
02

EQUIPMENT
WOK / PAN

MINUTES
20

DIFFICULTY
4/10

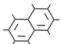

NUTRITIONAL INFORMATION:

587 CALORIES | 07 G CARBS | 44 G FAT | 40 G PROTEIN

INGREDIENTS

- **17.5 oz** beef strips *(500 g)*
- **1 tbsp** coconut oil
- **2 tbsp** sesame oil
- **1** carrot
- **1/2** red onion
- **1** zucchini

- **2** garlic cloves
- small handful basil
- **1/2 cup** coconut milk
- **1 tsp** paprika
- **1** beef stock cube
- **1 oz** cashews *(30g)*

PROCEDURE

Pre chop all the vegetables. Cut the zucchini into long strips, and the carrot into small diced pieces.

Add the coconut oil to the pan and heat up the oil with the ground garlic cloves and ginger. Next, add in the red onion. cook for about 3 mins.

Add the carrot to the pan, and 2 mins afterwards add the rest of the vegetables.

Remove from the frying pan and put onto a seperate plate. Add the beef strips to the pan and cook until lightly brown using the left over oil.

Add the vegetables back into the pan along with the coconut milk, stock and basil. Bring the pan down to a low simmer, add the cashews *(optional)* and let it cook for 5 mins.

Place into bowls and serve!

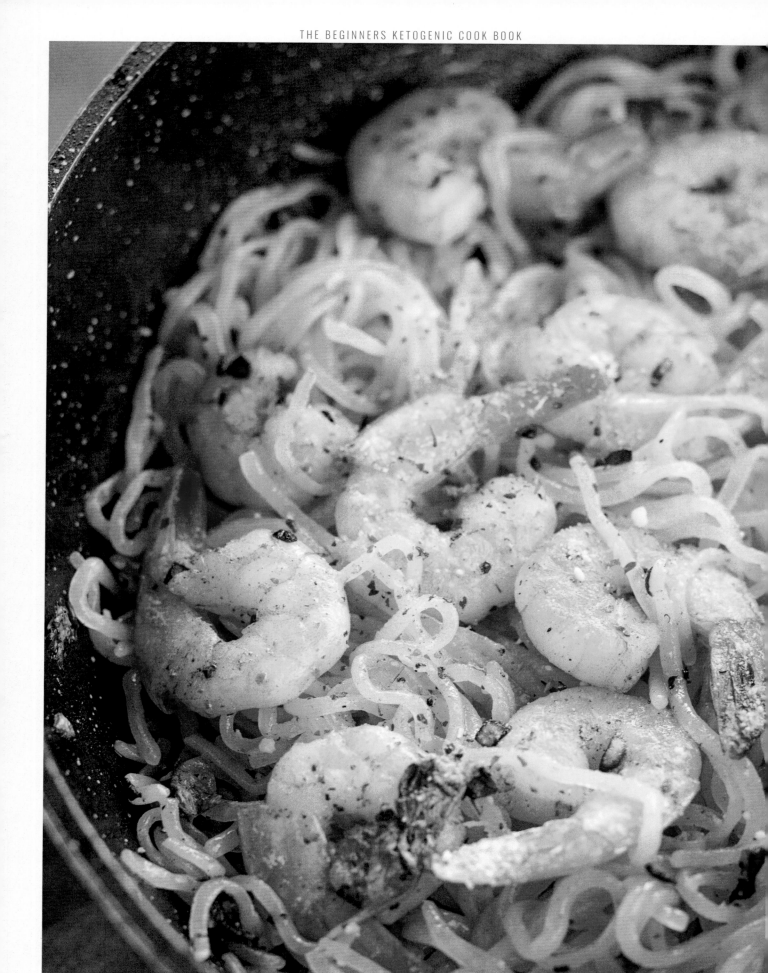

SHRIMP SCAMPI

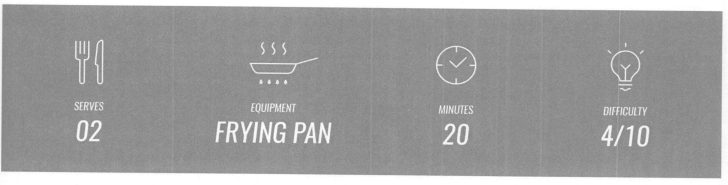

SERVES
02

EQUIPMENT
FRYING PAN

MINUTES
20

DIFFICULTY
4/10

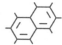

NUTRITIONAL INFORMATION:

489 CALORIES | **02 G CARBS** | **41 G FAT** | **25 G PROTEIN**

INGREDIENTS

- **10 oz** peeled shrimp *(300g)*
- **2** packets shirataki noodles
- **3** cloves garlic
- **6 tbsp** olive oil

- **2 tsp** white wine vinegar
- **1 tbsp** water
- **2 tbsp** lemon juice

PROCEDURE

Heat up a frying pan, drain the Shirataki noodles and dry fry them for about 8 mins. The noodles will turn a white colour.

Remove the noodles and reduce the heat to medium.

Add the olive oil and garlic, cook until slightly brown.

Add the prawns and cook until they change colour to a reddish hew (*Or you could use pre-cooked shrimp*).

Add the noodles and the rest of the ingredients to the pan. Toss until warm and serve.

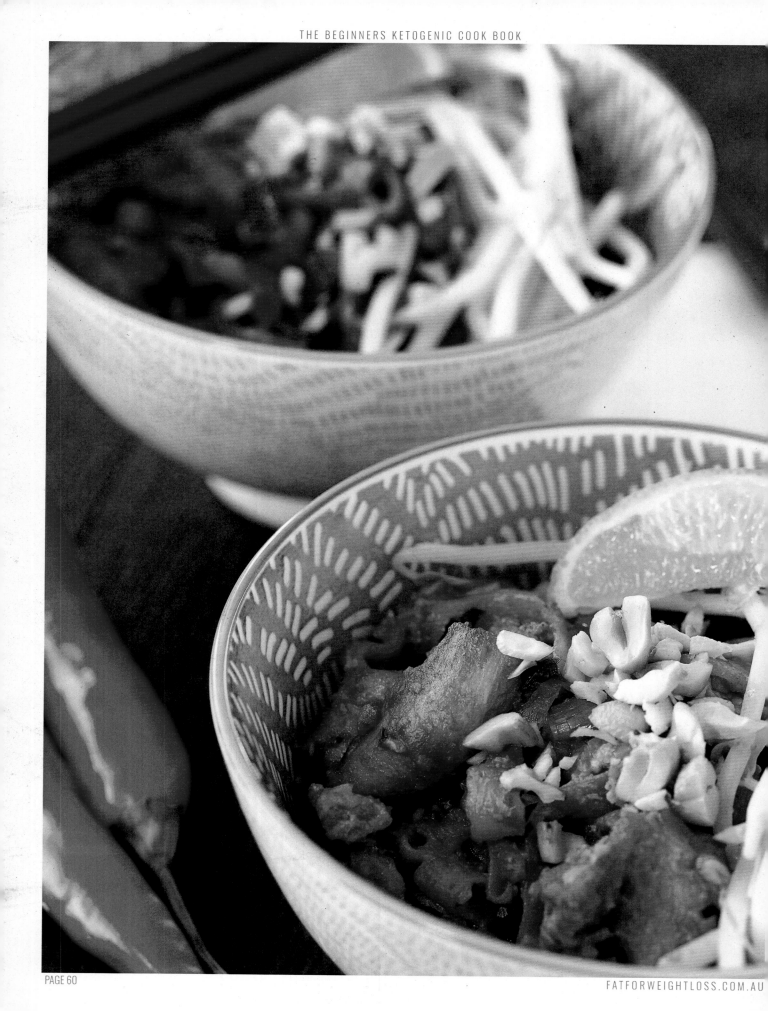

PAD THAI

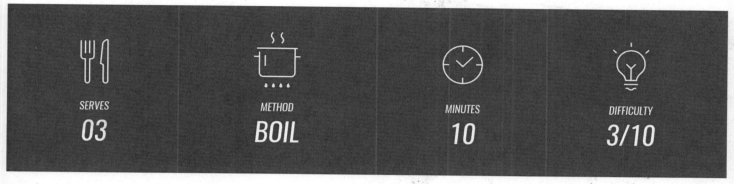

SERVES	METHOD	MINUTES	DIFFICULTY
03	BOIL	10	3/10

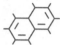

NUTRITIONAL INFORMATION:

490 CALORIES | **07 G CARBS** | **36 G FAT** | **23 G PROTEIN**

INGREDIENTS

- **2 tbsp** coriander *(cilantro)*
- **3** shallots *(green onions, chopped)*
- **2** eggs
- **2** packets shirataki noodles
- **3** chicken thighs
- **4 tbsp** coconut oil
- **4 oz** mung bean sprouts
- **2 tbsp** chopped nuts

SAUCE
- **1 ½ tbsp** sambal olek
- **1 ½ tsp** minced garlic
- **1 tbsp** peanut butter (organic)
- **1 tsp** rice wine vinegar
- **1 tsp** natvia (stevia)
- **1/2** lime juice
- **1 ½ tbsp** ketchup (no sugar)

- **1/2 tsp** worcestershire sauce
- **3 tbsp** fish sauce

PROCEDURE

Mix all the sauce ingredients together in a bowl with a fork.

Heat up a frying pan, cook the chicken for 5-10 mins with the coconut oil. Remove and set aside.

Rinse out the noodles. Heat up a frying pan and dry fry them for 5 mins. Reduce the heat and add the eggs.

Begin to scramble.

Add the sauce, chicken and the remaining ingredients into the pan. Toss until combined.

Serve and enjoy!

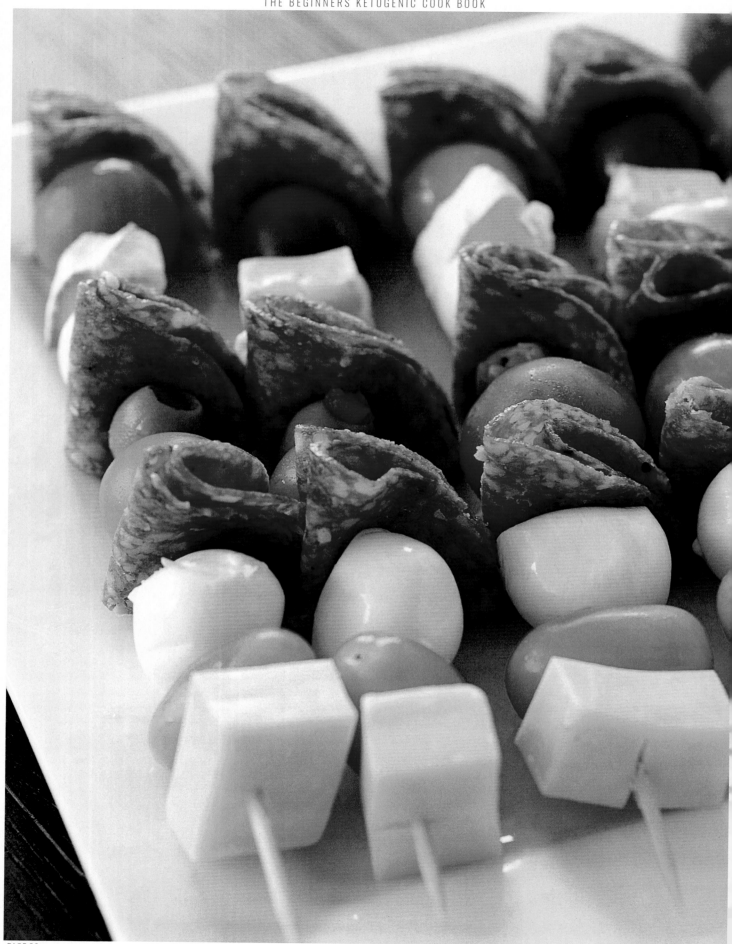

CHEESE AND SALAMI KEBABS

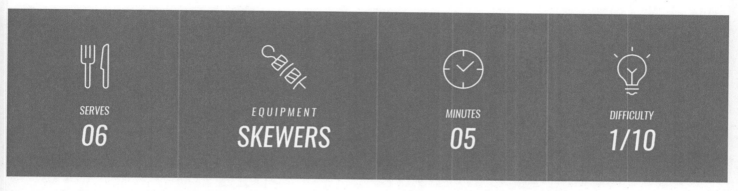

SERVES
06

EQUIPMENT
SKEWERS

MINUTES
05

DIFFICULTY
1/10

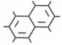

NUTRITIONAL INFORMATION:

299 CALORIES | 02 G CARBS | 24 G FAT | 20 G PROTEIN

INGREDIENTS

- **7 oz** cheddar cheese *(200 g)*
- **7 oz** bocconi *(200 g)*
- **3.5 oz** mild salami *(100 g)*

- **2 oz** olives *(50g)*
- **3.5 oz** tomatoes *(100 g)*
- **2 oz** camembert *(50 g)*

PROCEDURE

Spear all the ingredients onto kebab sticks and enjoy!

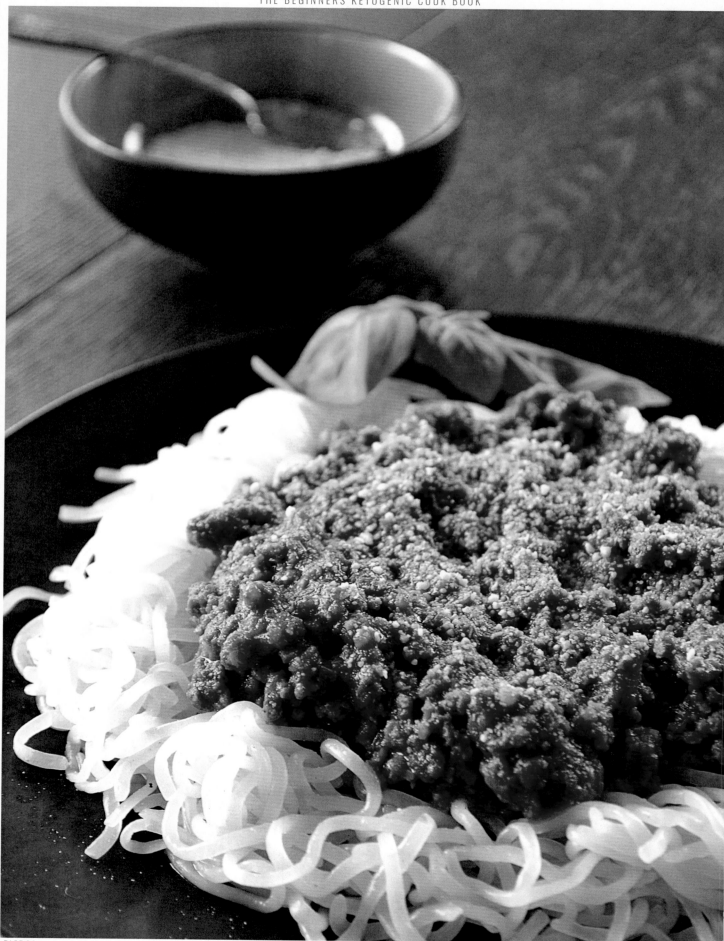

SPAGHETTI BOLOGNESE

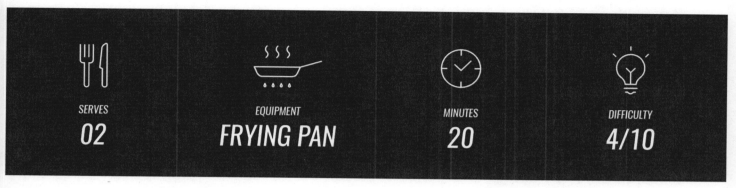

SERVES	EQUIPMENT	MINUTES	DIFFICULTY
02	FRYING PAN	20	4/10

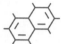

NUTRITIONAL INFORMATION:

238 CALORIES | **04 G CARBS** | **13 G FAT** | **25 G PROTEIN**

INGREDIENTS

- **1/2 cup** passata sauce (*tomato puree*)
- **1/2 cup** diced tomatoes
- **2 cups** ground beef (*500g / 17 oz*)
- **1 tsp** worcestershire sauce

- **1 tsp** italian herbs
- **1 tsp** garlic
- **1 packet** miracle noodles
- **1 tbsp** parmesan cheese

PROCEDURE

Add the Mince into a frying pan (*1 lb*) and cook until slightly brown. Add the Garlic, Worcestershire sauce and Italian Herbs and cook for 1 min.

Pour in the Passata sauce and diced tomatoes, simmering for 10 Mins.

In this time, take the miracle noodles and drain the water (*I used a sieve*). Wash them slightly and place them inside a light cloth to completely drain the water out.

In a second frying pan, dry fry the noodles for about 2 mins. This will cook the noodles and remove the excess water.

You can either serve with the noodles plain, or mix the noodles into the sauce. Top with parmesan cheese, sever and enjoy!

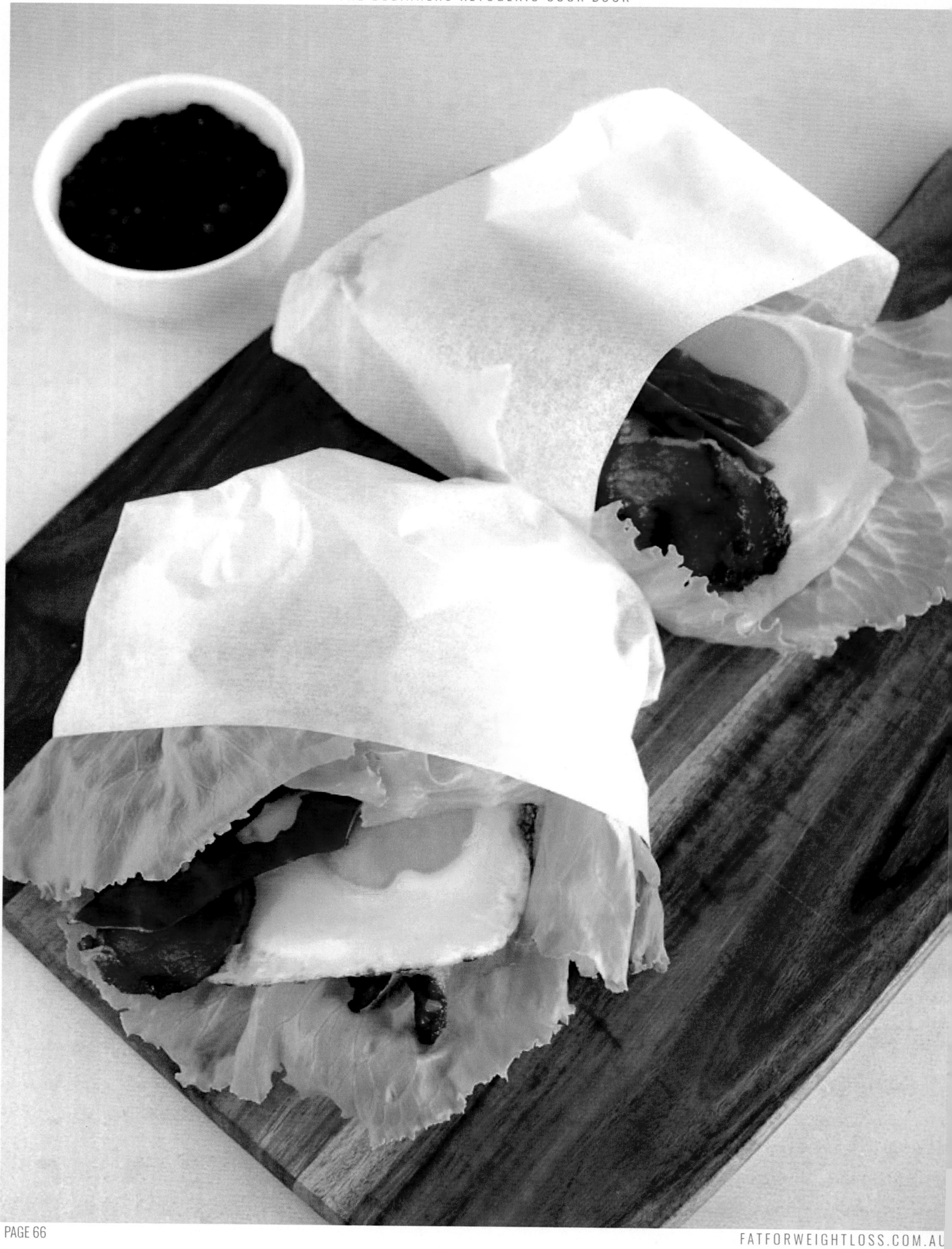

BACON AND EGG LET TUCE WRAP

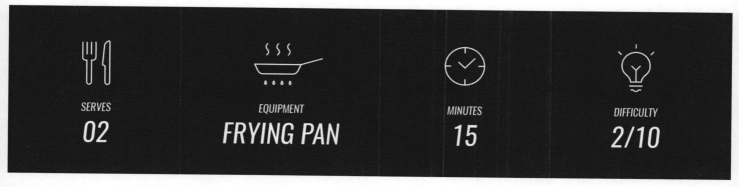

SERVES	EQUIPMENT	MINUTES	DIFFICULTY
02	FRYING PAN	15	2/10

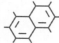

NUTRITIONAL INFORMATION:

605 CALORIES | **04 G CARBS** | **43 G FAT** | **40 G PROTEIN**

INGREDIENTS

- **2** lettuce leaves
- **3** slices bacon (*100g / 3.5 oz*)
- **2** eggs fried
- **1/2 cup** red cabbage

PROCEDURE

Heat up a frying pan, cook bacon until crispy.

In a seperate pan, cook the eggs until your liking.

Cut each lettuce leaf off at the stalk and place the ingredients inside. Should make 2 burgers.

Wrap together and eat with keto confidence!

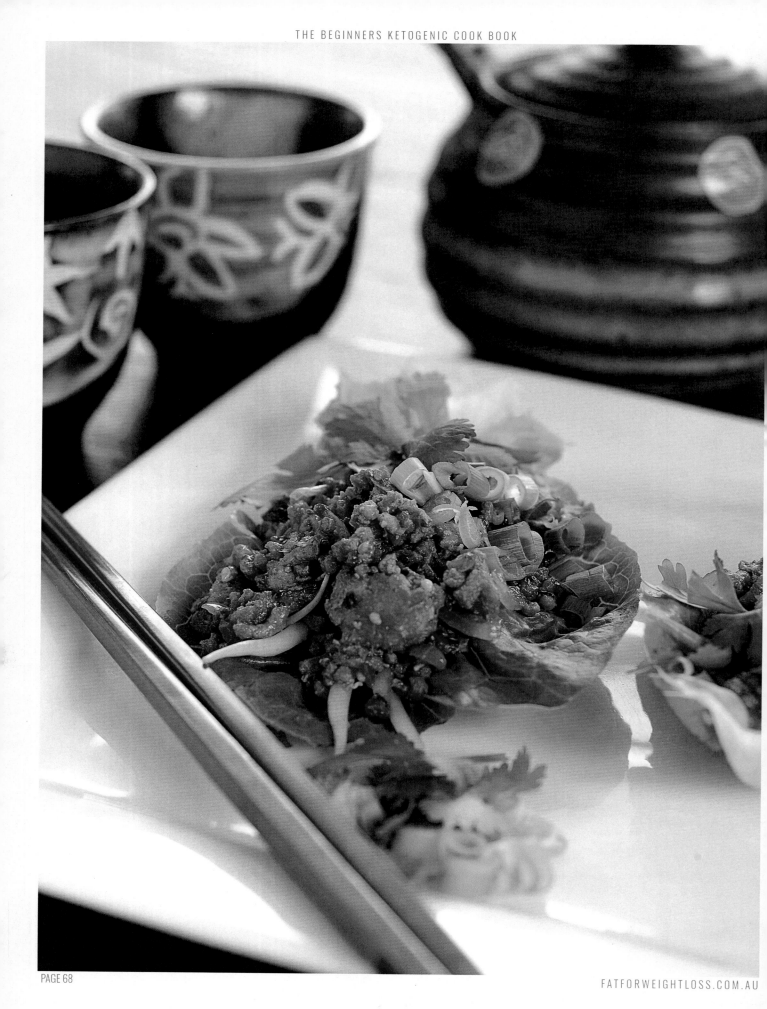

SAN CHOY BAU

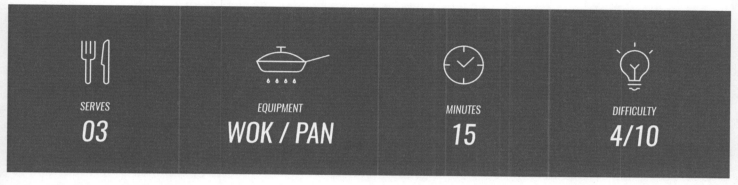

SERVES
03

EQUIPMENT
WOK / PAN

MINUTES
15

DIFFICULTY
4/10

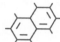

NUTRITIONAL INFORMATION:

267 CALORIES | 07 G CARBS | 11 G FAT | 35 G PROTEIN

INGREDIENTS

- **2** garlic cloves crushed
- **2 cm** piece ginger finely grated
- **17 oz** pork mince *(500 g)*
- **2 tbsp** soy sauce
- **2** shallots thinly sliced

- **1/2** lime juiced
- **1 tsp** sesame oil
- **1 cup** beansprouts trimmed
- **12** large lettuce leaves
- **1/4 cup** fresh coriander leaves

PROCEDURE

Heat wok *(or frying pan)* over high heat until hot. Add sesame seed oil, garlic, ginger and pork. fry for 2 to 3 minutes or until pork just changes colour.

Add soy sauce and onions, 2 teaspoons of lime juice.

Fry for 3 minutes or until heated through. Stir in beansprouts.

Spoon pork mixture into lettuce leaves. Sprinkle with coriander. Serve and Enjoy!

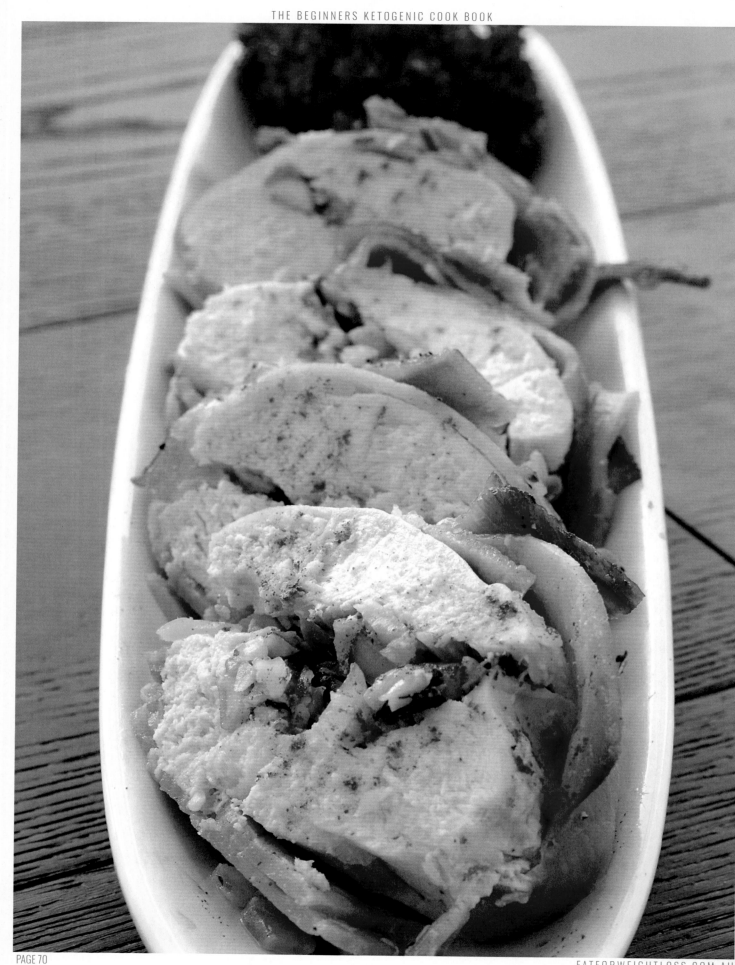

BACON WRAPPED STUFFED CHICKEN

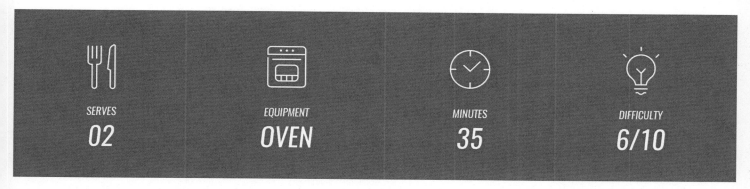

SERVES
02

EQUIPMENT
OVEN

MINUTES
35

DIFFICULTY
6/10

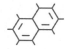

NUTRITIONAL INFORMATION:

484 CALORIES | **07 G CARBS** | **47 G FAT** | **24 G PROTEIN**

INGREDIENTS

- **1** chicken breast
- **6** slices bacon *(300g / 10.5 oz)*
- **1** handful cashews *(50 g / 1.5 oz)*
- **3 tbsps** sesame seed oil
- **1 tsp** coriander

PROCEDURE

Slice the chicken breast in half *(as if you where to butterfly cut)*.

Chop up nuts finely, also chop the herbs and add the sesame seed oil to a small bowl.

Fill the chicken with the stuffing, and carefully wrap 5 slices of bacon around lengthwise, keeping 1 slice of bacon to cover from top to bottom.

Place on a baking tray, cook at 180 C *(375 F)* for 30 mins. Depending on how large the chicken breast is, you might need an extra few minutes for the chicken to cook through thoroughly.

Remove from the oven, and let it rest before you cut it.

Enjoy!

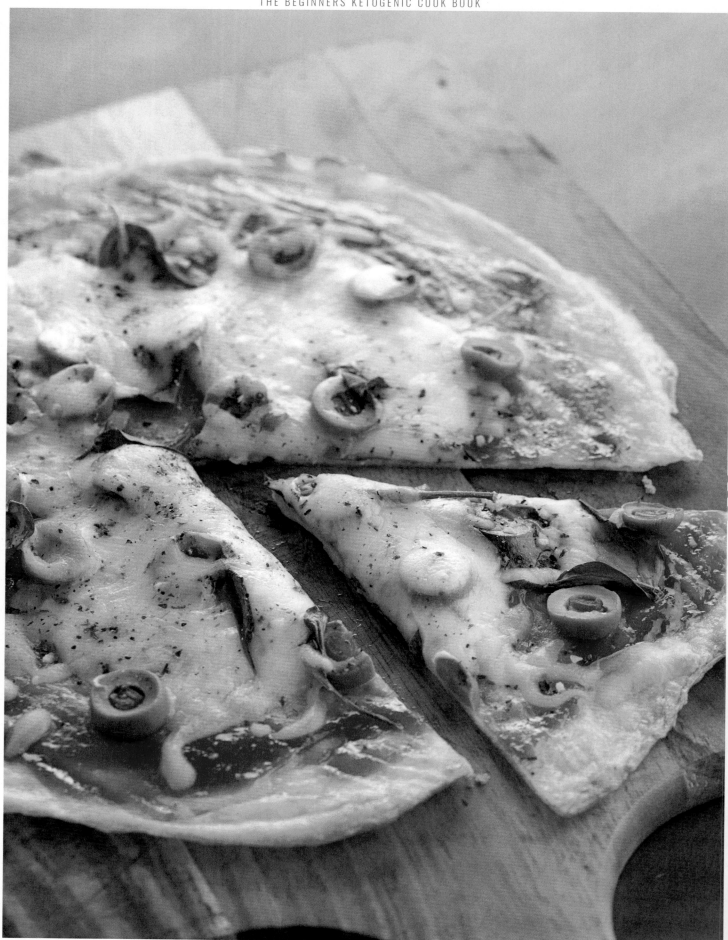

FATHEAD PIZZA (CHEESE PIZZA)

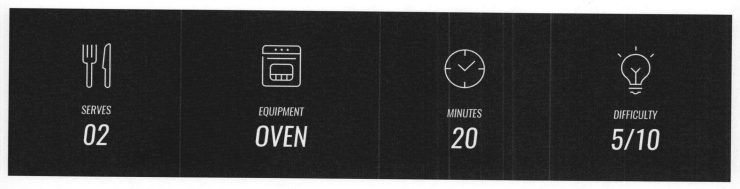

SERVES	EQUIPMENT	MINUTES	DIFFICULTY
02	OVEN	20	5/10

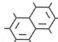

NUTRITIONAL INFORMATION:

500 CALORIES | **05 G CARBS** | **38 G FAT** | **30 G PROTEIN**

INGREDIENTS

BASE
- **1 cup** mozzarella cheese
- **1 tbsp** almond flour
- **1 tbsp** cream cheese
- **1 large** egg
- **1/2 tsp** salt
- **1/2 tsp** pepper

TOPPINGS
- **1 cup** mozzarella cheese
- **1/4 cup** tomato sauce
- **16** slices pepperoni
- **1 tsp** dried oregano seasoning
- **1 tbsp** olives *(optional)*

PROCEDURE

Preheat the oven to 390 F *(200 C)* Put the mozzarella cheese into a microwave safe bowl and microwave for 90 secs.

Mix in the rest of the base ingredients with a fork.

Roll out with a rolling pin into round slices *(you can use a bowl and a knife to make perfect circles)*.

Put the base in the oven for 7 mins, flip the base and cook the other side for 3 mins.

Take the pizza out of the oven. Using a tablespoon, smother the pizza base with the tomato sauce. Add the pepperoni, Cover in cheese and place in the oven for another 10 mins.

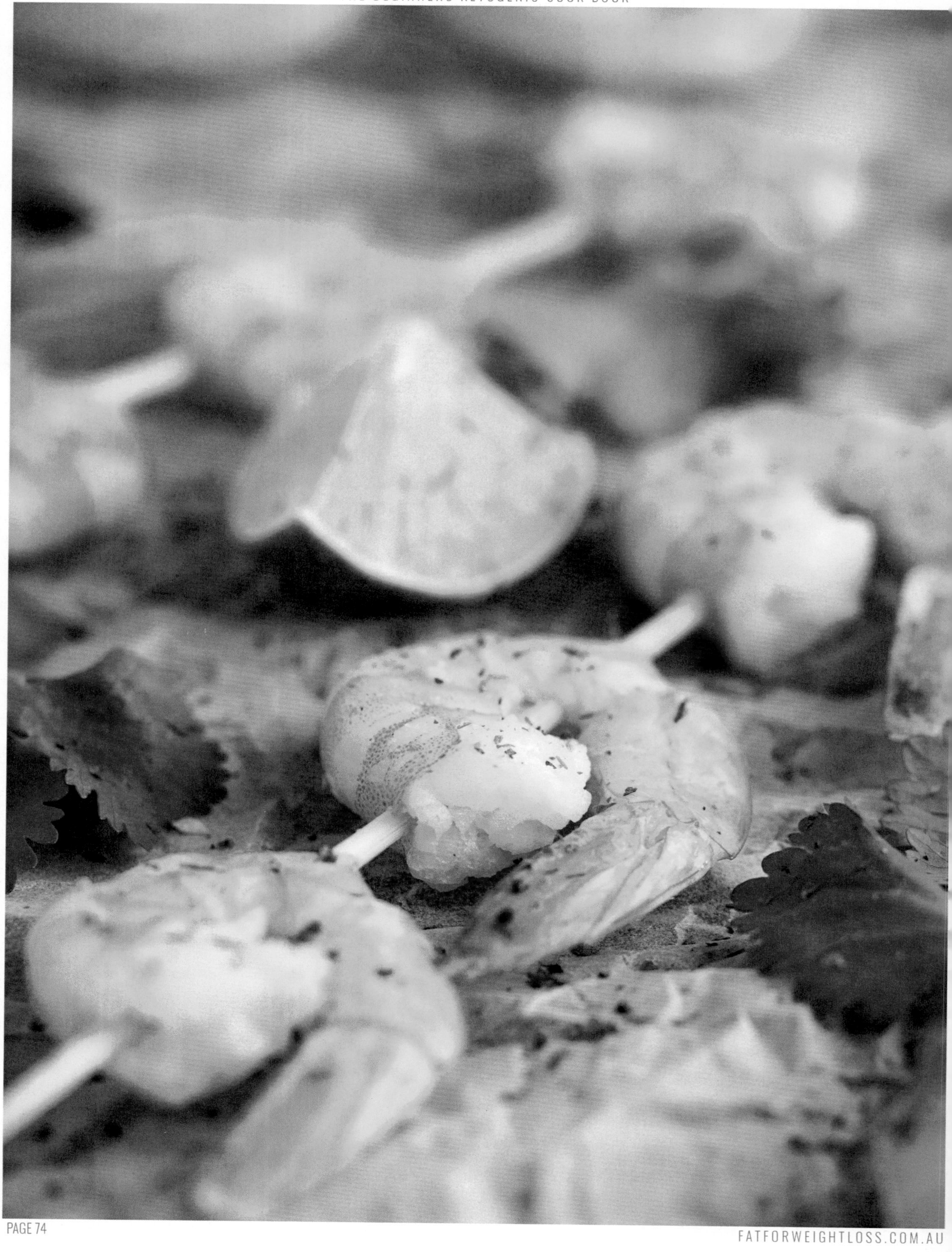

SHRIMP SKEWERS

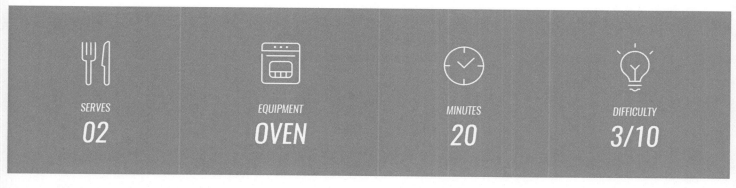

SERVES
02

EQUIPMENT
OVEN

MINUTES
20

DIFFICULTY
3/10

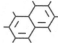

NUTRITIONAL INFORMATION:

365 CALORIES | **02 G CARBS** | **36 G FAT** | **30 G PROTEIN**

INGREDIENTS

- **5 oz** shrimp (*150 g*)
- **1 tbsp** olive oil
- **3 tbsp** butter
- **3** cloves garlic

- **1/4 tsp** salt
- **1/2** lime
- **1 tbsp** cilantro for garnish (coriander)
- **6** short bamboo skewers, soaked in water.

PROCEDURE

Heat up the grill. Thread the shrimp onto the bamboo skewers. Cook the shrimp for 10-15 mins, basting with olive oil at regular intervals.

Melt the butter and garlic in a small saucepan. Once the shrimp has finished cooking, place on a plate or pan and cover with the garlic butter.

Cover with lime and salt, serve and enjoy!

SALMON WITH BASIL MAYONNAISE

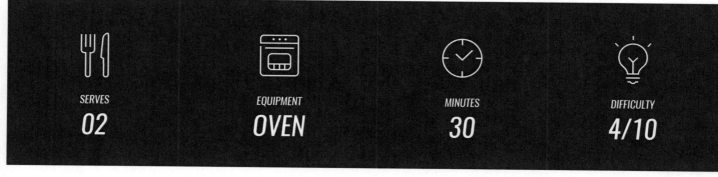

SERVES	EQUIPMENT	MINUTES	DIFFICULTY
02	OVEN	30	4/10

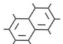

NUTRITIONAL INFORMATION:

315 CALORIES | 02 G CARBS | 25 G FAT | 22 G PROTEIN

INGREDIENTS

- **2** salmon fillet
- **2 tbsp** olive oil
- **1 tbsp** lemon juice
- **1/2 tsp** salt
- **1/2 tsp** pepper

BASIL MAYONNAISE
- **2 tbsp** basil
- **1/4 cup** olive oil
- **1** egg yolk
- **1/2 tbsp** lemon juice

PROCEDURE

Take 2 square sheets of aluminium foil, and place each piece of salmon in each, dividing the remaining ingredients between the two pieces.

Cover the salmon with the foil by wrapping the ends.

Bake in the oven at 350 F (*180 C)* for 25 mins.

While the salmon is cooking, in a blender, mix the basil mayonnaise ingredients together until smooth.

Serve with the salmon. Enjoy!

SRIRACHA SALMON

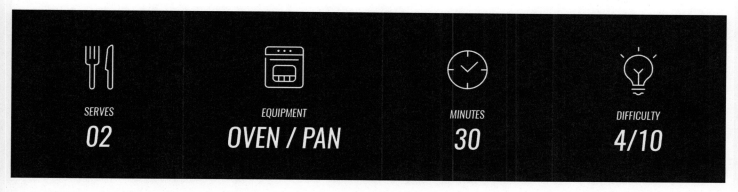

SERVES
02

EQUIPMENT
OVEN / PAN

MINUTES
30

DIFFICULTY
4/10

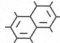

NUTRITIONAL INFORMATION:

334 CALORIES | **08 G CARBS** | **25 G FAT** | **25 G PROTEIN**

INGREDIENTS

- **1 tbsp** sriracha sauce
- **2** limes
- **2** salmon fillets
- **1 tbsp** sesame seed oil

- **1/4 tsp** salt
- **1/2** lime
- **1 tbsp** cilantro for garnish (coriander)
- **6** short bamboo skewers, soaked in water.

PROCEDURE

Preheat the oven to 320 F *(160 C)* Heat a frying pan and sear the salmon fillets skin down for 2 mins.

Combine the Sriracha sauce, 2 Tbsps. of lime juice and the sesame seed oil into a small bowl.

Remove the salmon from the frying pan, place each piece of salmon individually inside aluminium foil *(shiny side up)* and baste with the sauce. Place in the oven.

Cook for 15-20 mins. Enjoy!

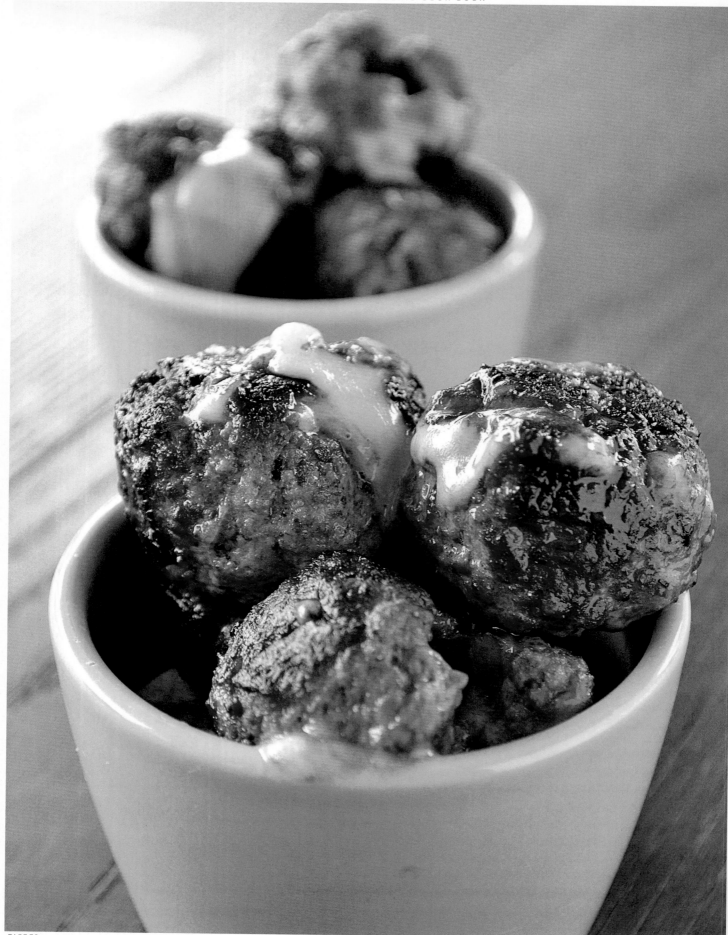

CHEESE MEATBALLS

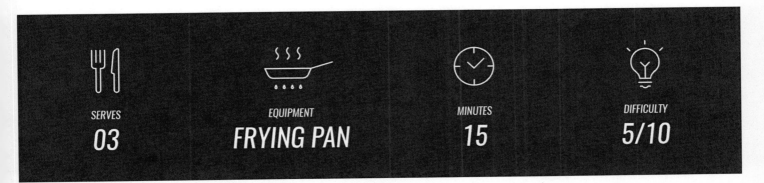

SERVES	EQUIPMENT	MINUTES	DIFFICULTY
03	FRYING PAN	15	5/10

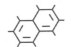

NUTRITIONAL INFORMATION:

440 CALORIES | **02 G CARBS** | **28 G FAT** | **46 G PROTEIN**

INGREDIENTS

- **1 lb** ground beef (*500g*)
- **3.5 oz** mozzarella cheese (100g)
- **3 tbsp** parmesan cheese
- **1 tsp** garlic powder
- **1/2 tsp** salt
- **1/2 tsp** pepper

PROCEDURE

Cut the cheese into cubes (*1cm by 1cm*).

Mix the dry ingredients with the ground beef.

Wrap the cubes of cheese in beef (*ground beef should make about 9 Balls*).

Pan fry the meatballs. (*Cover with a lid to capture the heat all around*).

Alternitvely, you can cook these in the oven at 180C (*355F*) for 25 mins.

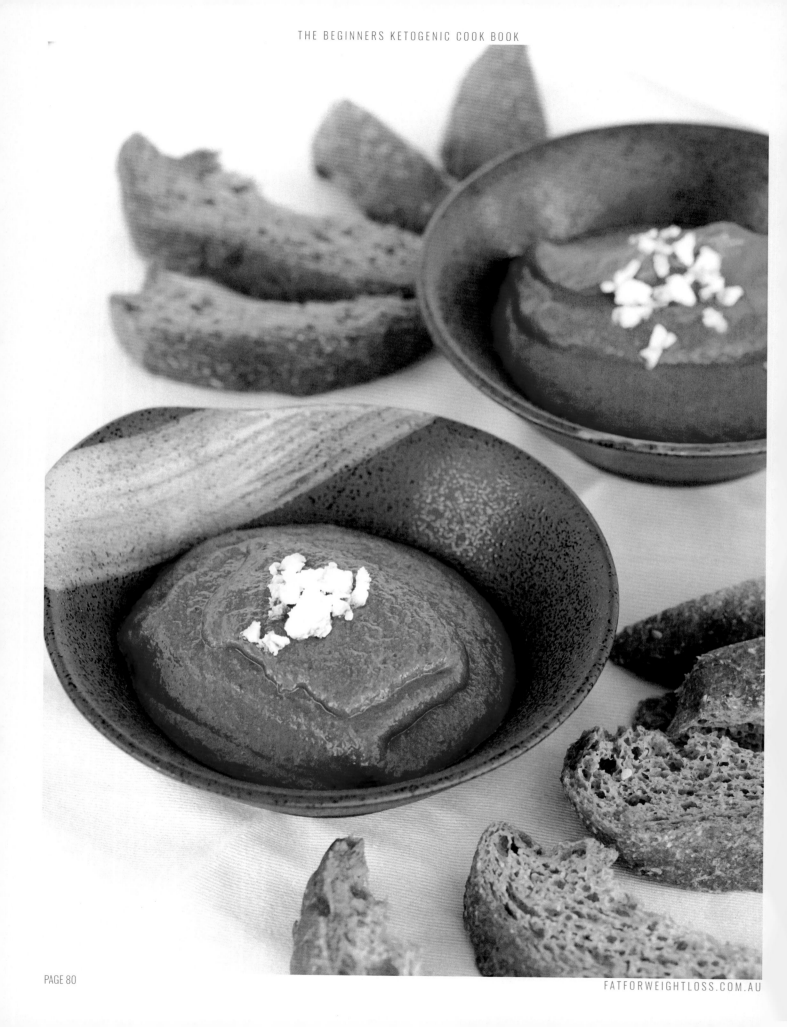

ROAST BEETROOT AND FETA DIP

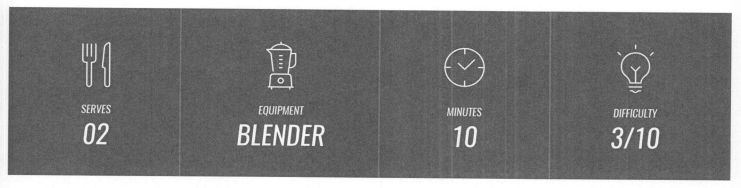

SERVES	EQUIPMENT	MINUTES	DIFFICULTY
02	BLENDER	10	3/10

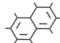

NUTRITIONAL INFORMATION:

343 CALORIES | **03 G CARBS** | **21 G FAT** | **20 G PROTEIN**

INGREDIENTS

- **1** large beetroot
- **3.5 oz** danish feta cheese *(100g)*
- **2 oz** olive oil *(60 ml)*
- **1 ½** garlic cloves
- **1/2** tsp salt
- **1/2** tsp pepper

PROCEDURE

Put all the ingredients into a mixer, and blend until smooth.

Serve with oven roasted keto bread rolls.

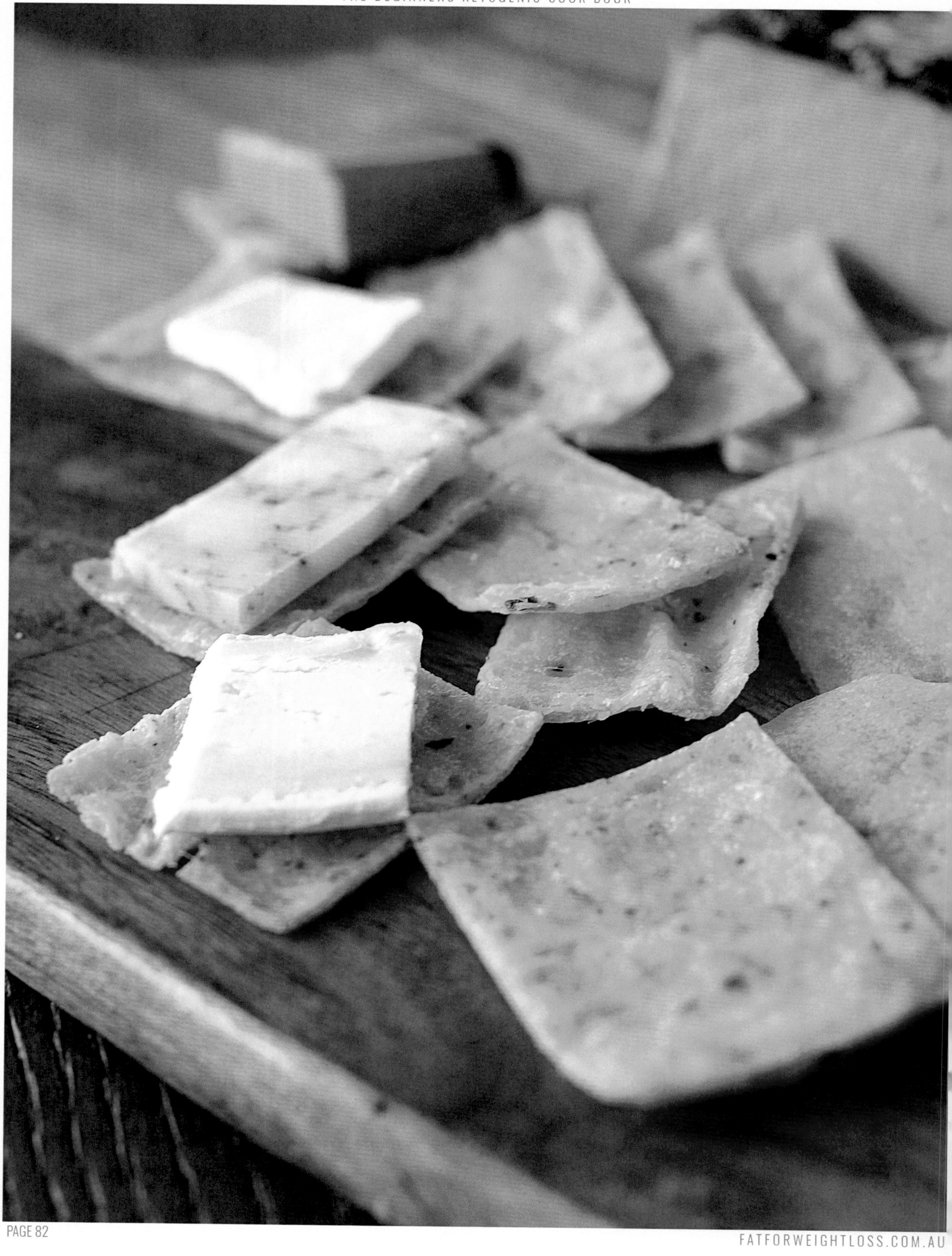

FATHEAD CRACKERS

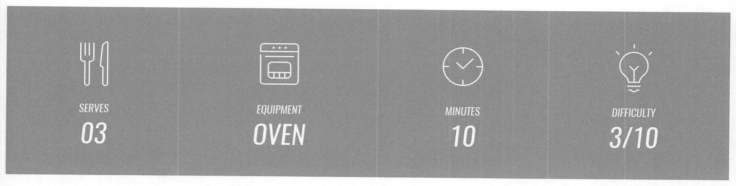

SERVES
03

EQUIPMENT
OVEN

MINUTES
10

DIFFICULTY
3/10

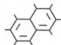

NUTRITIONAL INFORMATION:

334 CALORIES | **02 G CARBS** | **17 G FAT** | **16 G PROTEIN**

INGREDIENTS

- **1 cup** mozzarella cheese
- **1 tbsp** almond flour
- **1 egg**

PROCEDURE

Preheat the oven to 390 ° F *(200 ° C)*.

Put the mozzarella cheese into a microwave safe bowl and microwave for 90 secs.

Mix in the remaining the ingredients. Knead with your hands.

Roll out with a rolling pin into a large flat thin area.

Put the crackers in the oven for 10 mins, and continue cooking until crispy in 5 min increments.

Remove from oven, cut into cracker sized pieces and return to the oven for another 5 mins.

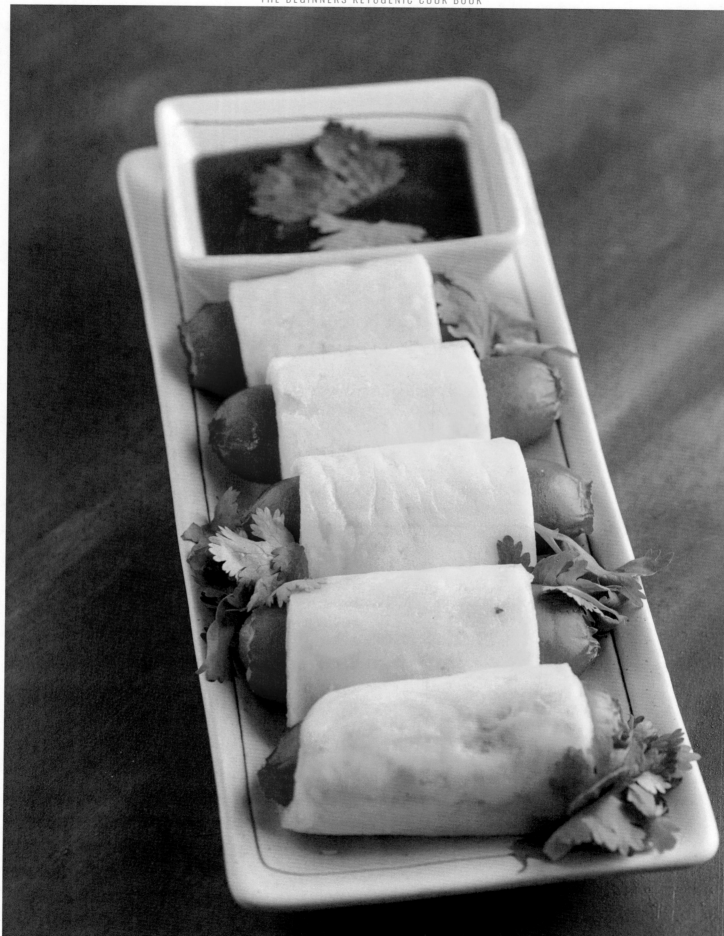

PIGS IN BLANKETS

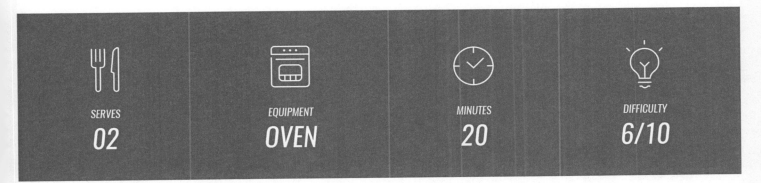

SERVES
02

EQUIPMENT
OVEN

MINUTES
20

DIFFICULTY
6/10

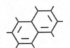

NUTRITIONAL INFORMATION:

363 CALORIES | 04 G CARBS | 27 G FAT | 25 G PROTEIN

INGREDIENTS

- **5** cocktail hotdogs
- **1 cup** mozzarella cheese
- **1 tbsp** almond meal
- **1** large egg
- **1/2 tsp** salt

PROCEDURE

Preheat the oven to 355 ° F *(180 ° C)*.

Put the mozzarella cheese into a microwave safe bowl and microwave for 60 secs.

Mix in the remaining the almond flour and the eggs with a fork.

Roll out between two sheets of parchment paper with a rolling pin into a large flat thin area.

Put the dough in the oven for 7 mins.

Bring a pot of water to the boil. Begin to boil the hotdogs.

Remove the dough from the oven and cut into long strips not quite as wide as the hotdogs. Roll the hotdogs in the dough until once around. Return to the oven and bake for another 10 mins.

Enjoy!

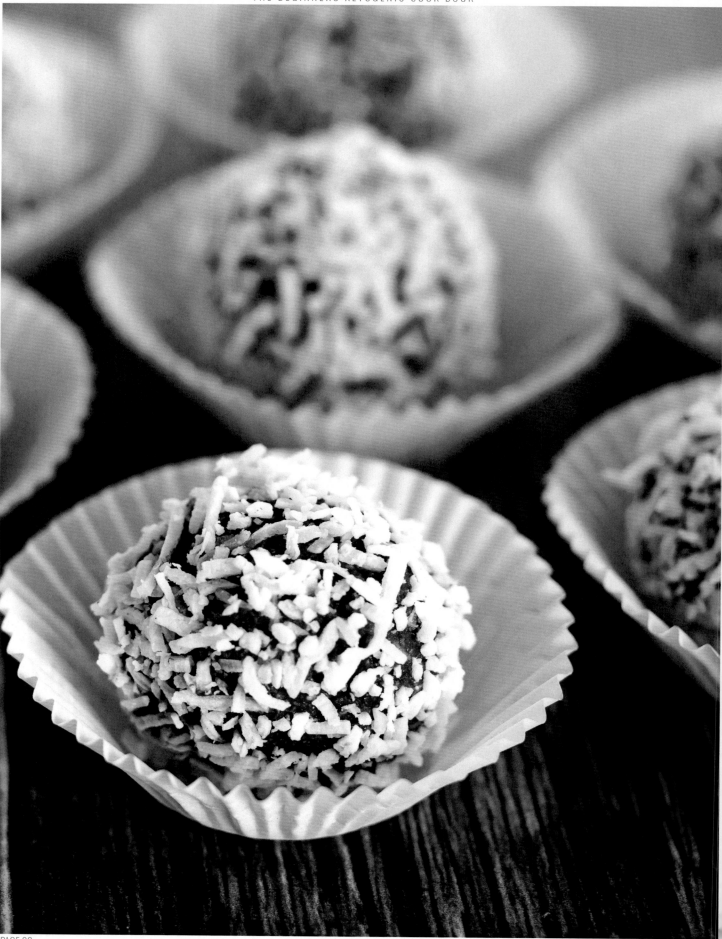

CHOCOLATE COCONUT FAT BOMBS (FAT TIES)

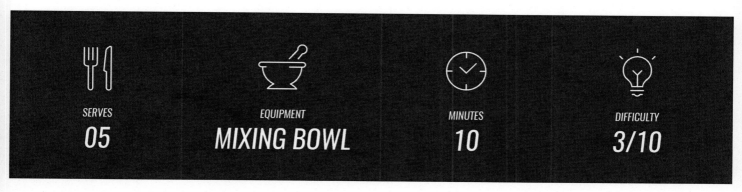

SERVES
05

EQUIPMENT
MIXING BOWL

MINUTES
10

DIFFICULTY
3/10

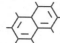

NUTRITIONAL INFORMATION:

282 CALORIES | **06 G CARBS** | **26 G FAT** | **06 G PROTEIN**

INGREDIENTS

- **1/4 cup** coconut oil
- **1/4 cup** cocoa powder
- **4 tbsp** peanut butter
- **6 tbsp** chia seeds
- **2 tbsp** heavy cream

- **1/4 cup** almond flour
- **1/4 cup** unsweetened shredded coconut
- **2 tsp** sugar subsitute
- **1 tsp** vanilla extract

PROCEDURE

Mix all the dry ingredients in a bowl with the coconut oil – This will eventually form a paste type consistency.

Add the peanut butter and make sure the mixture stays a relatively sticky consistency.

Add the vanilla essence and sugar substitute to the mix.

Put about 1/4 cup of extra shredded coconut on a plate, form balls with the mixture and roll those fatties.

Keep refrigerated

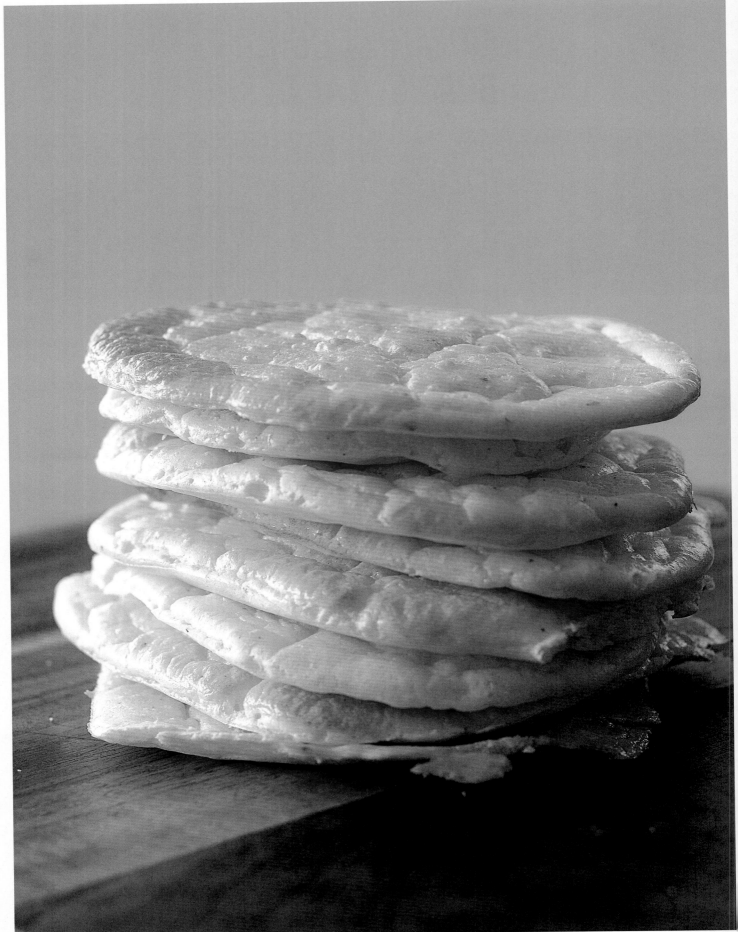

CLOUD BREAD

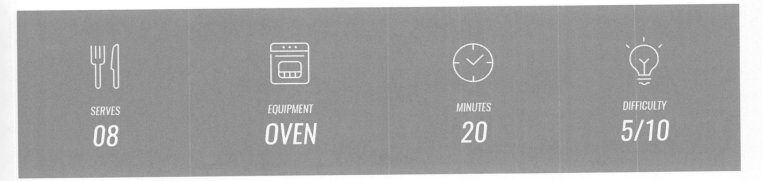

SERVES	EQUIPMENT	MINUTES	DIFFICULTY
08	OVEN	20	5/10

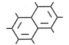

NUTRITIONAL INFORMATION PER 1 SLICE:

122 CALORIES | **01 G CARBS** | **10 G FAT** | **07G PROTEIN**

INGREDIENTS

- **4** large eggs
- **1/2 tsp** cream of tartar
- **1/4 cup** cream cheese
- **1/2 tsp** salt

PROCEDURE

Crack the eggs and separate the whites from the yolks. Put all the whites into a bowl and whisk with an electric mixer for 1 - 2 mins.

Add the Cream Of Tartar and whisk again for another 1 min. The mixture should start making soft peaks.

In another bowl, add the yolks and the cream cheese and mix on high until well combined. Gently fold this mixture into the egg whites.

Spoon out the final mixture onto a tray lined with baking paper. They do fluff up a bit in the oven so leave enough space to breathe!

Put in the oven on 180 ° c *(375 ° F)* for 15-20 mins until slightly golden brown on top. Serve and enjoy!

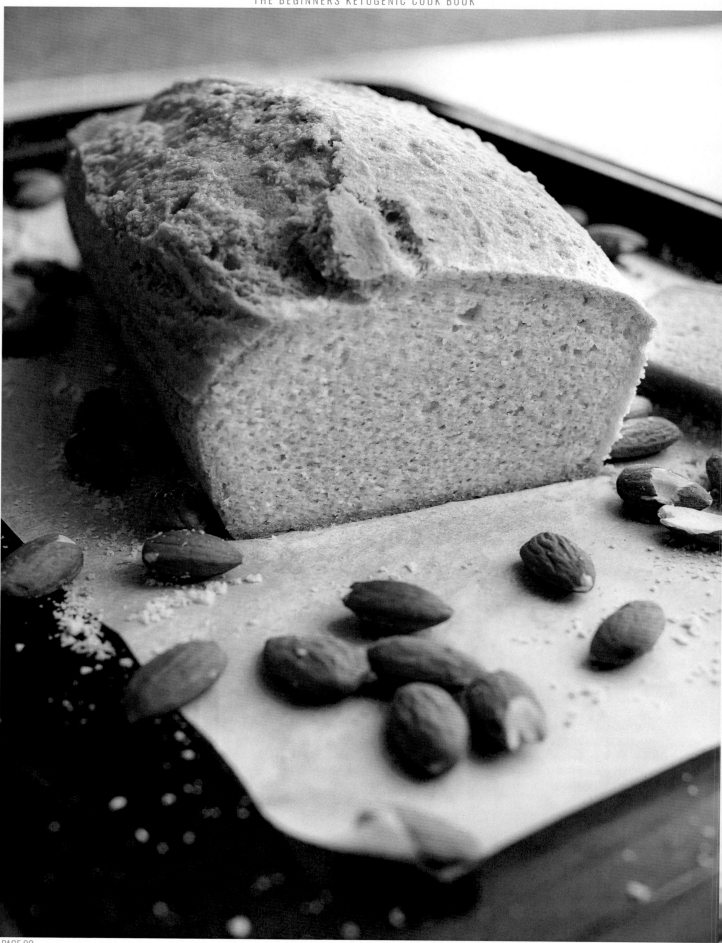

KETOGENIC BREAD

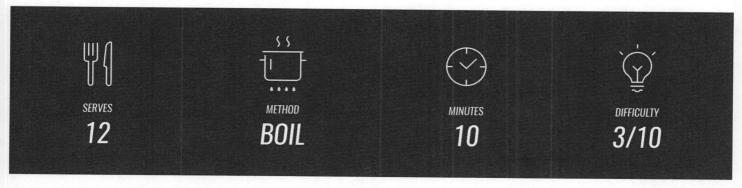

SERVES	METHOD	MINUTES	DIFFICULTY
12	BOIL	10	3/10

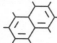

NUTRITIONAL INFORMATION:

278 CALORIES | 02 G CARBS | 28 G FAT | 09 G PROTEIN

INGREDIENTS

- **1/2 cup** butter (*melted*)
- **3 tbsp** coconut oil
- **8** eggs
- **1 tsp** baking powder

- **2 cup** almond flour
- **1/2 tsp** xanthium gum
- **1/2 tsp** salt

PROCEDURE

Preheat oven to 160 ° C (*350 ° F*).

Put the eggs into a bowl and beat for 1 - 2 mins on high.

Add coconut oil and melted butter to eggs, continue beating.

Add remaining ingredients. Will become quite thick.

Scrape into a loaf pan lined with baking paper.

Bake for 40 minutes. (*Remove once a skewer comes out of the middle clean*).

Allow to cool before slicing.

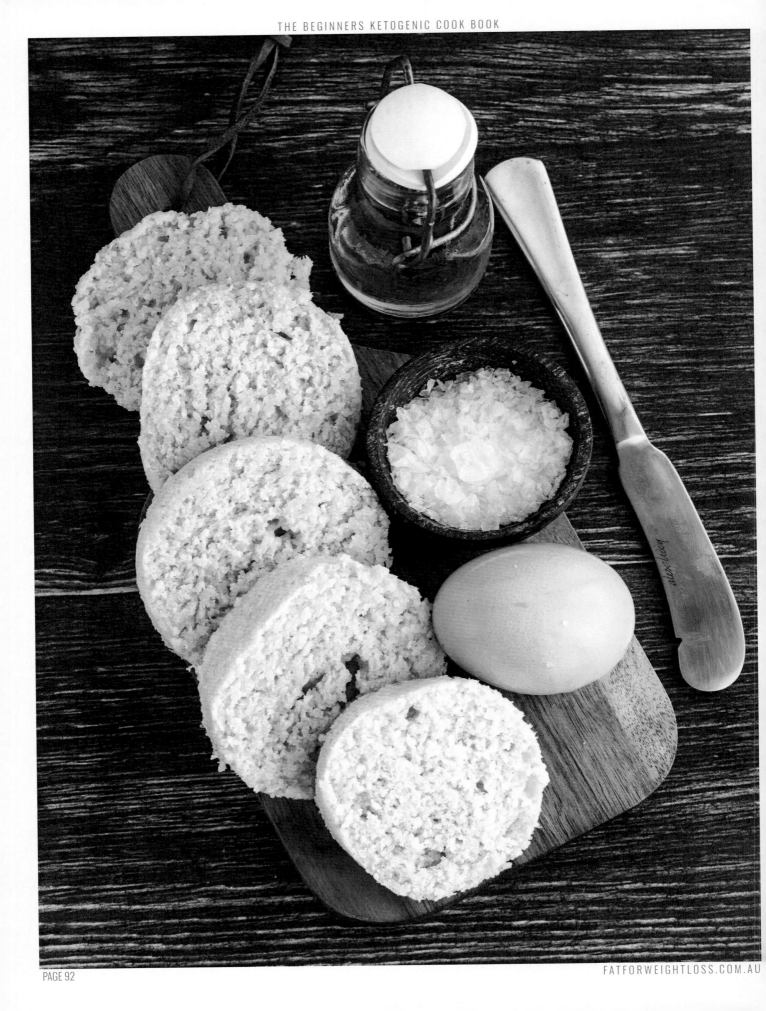

ALMOST INSTANT KETO BREAD

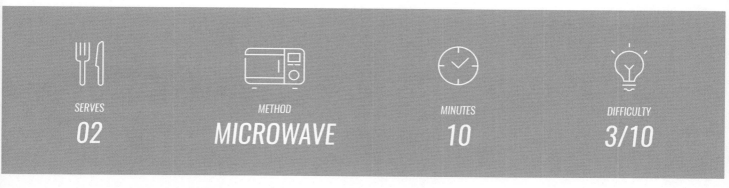

SERVES
02

METHOD
MICROWAVE

MINUTES
10

DIFFICULTY
3/10

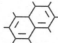

NUTRITIONAL INFORMATION:

160 CALORIES | **01 G CARBS** | **17 G FAT** | **6.5 G PROTEIN**

INGREDIENTS

- **1 tbsp** coconut flour
- **1/4 cup** almond flour
- **1 tbsp** coconut oil
- **1/2 tsp** baking powder
- **1 egg**

PROCEDURE

Place all the ingredients into a mug. Mix until combined with a fork. Microwave for 90 seconds.

Optionally, place ingredients in a small baking tray and cook for 10-15 mins at 375° F (*180° C).*

Cut and enjoy.

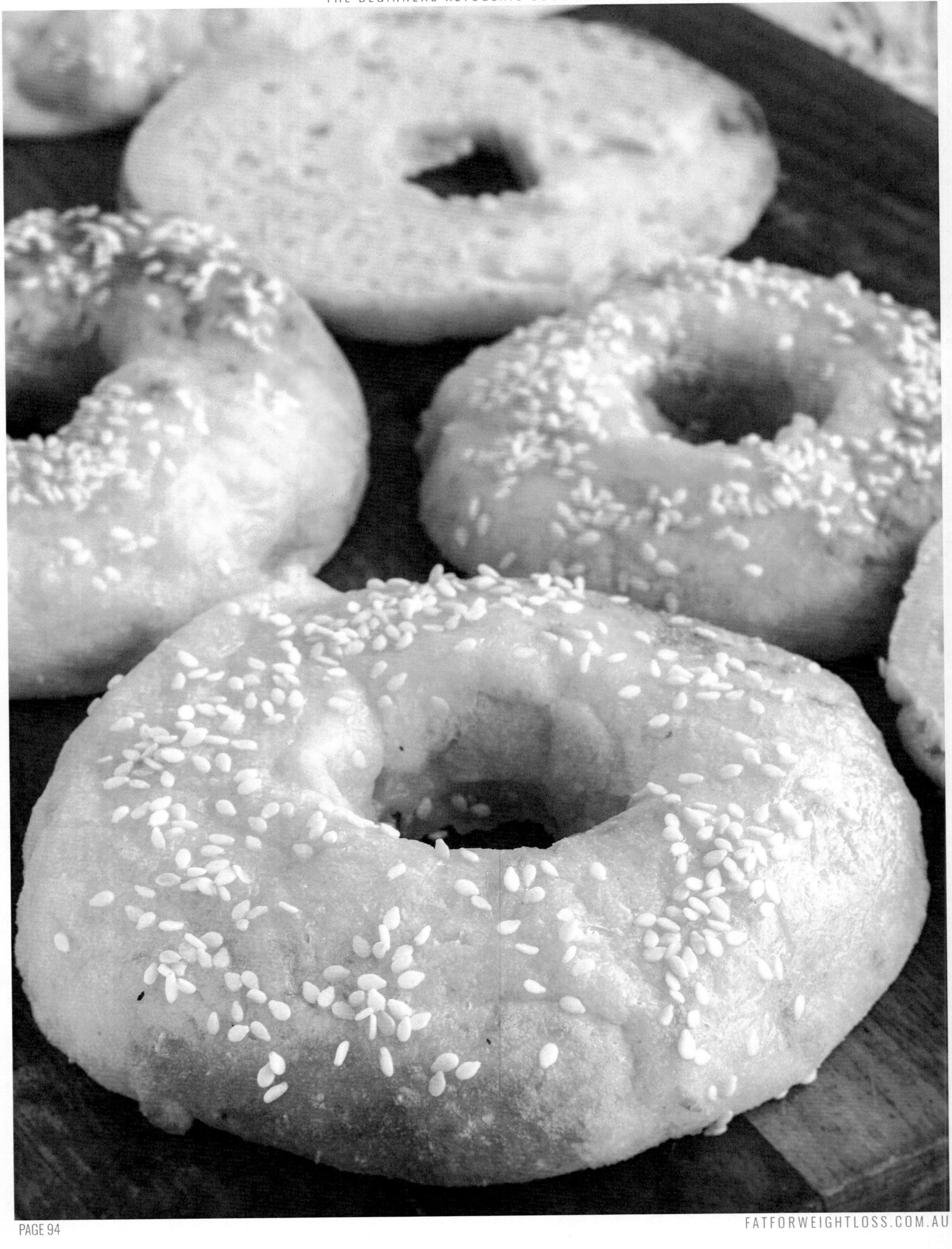

BAGELS

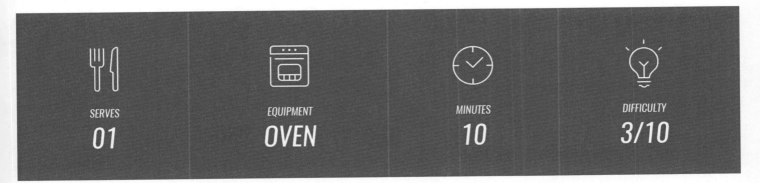

SERVES	EQUIPMENT	MINUTES	DIFFICULTY
01	OVEN	10	3/10

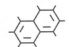

NUTRITIONAL INFORMATION PER BAGEL:

320 CALORIES | **05 G CARBS** | **24 G FAT** | **19 G PROTEIN**

INGREDIENTS

- **1 1/4 cups** almond meal
- **2 cups** mozzarella cheese
- **1/4 cup** cream cheese
- **2 tbsp** whey protien powder

- **1 tbsp** baking powder
- **2** large eggs
- **1 tbsp** sesame seeds

PROCEDURE

Preheat your oven to 180C (*355 F*).

Place the mozarella into a microwave safe bowl, and heat for 2 Mins (*You can do this in a double boiler if you don't have a microwave*).

Remove and mix in the cream cheese and 2 eggs. (*keep a little egg white for later to glaze the bagels*).

In a seperate bowl, Mix the almond flour, whey protien powder and baking powder together until well mixed together. Add this to the hot cheese mixture.

Make sure you mix the cheese and almond flour mixture very well. You don't want to see any clumps of almond flour in the mixture.

Cut the mixture in the bowl into 6 peices (*using three cuts. one in half, and two in diagonal directions*). Remove each of the 6 peices and roll into a 6 inch long sausage.

Get a baking tray, cover with partchment paper and place your sausage looking rolls onto the tray, and make them into circles, joining the edges togther with your fingers.

Using the left over egg white, brush each bagel and cover with sesame seeds. Place in the oven for 15 - 20 mins until just before it starts to turn brown. Remove from the oven, let cool, and enjoy.

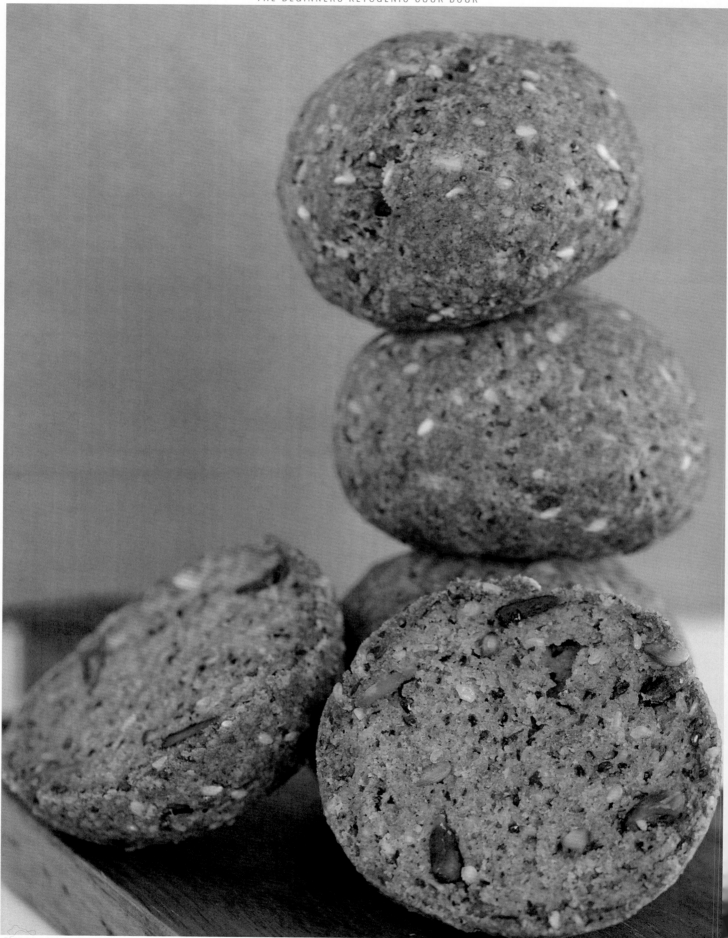

GRAIN FREE DINNER ROLLS

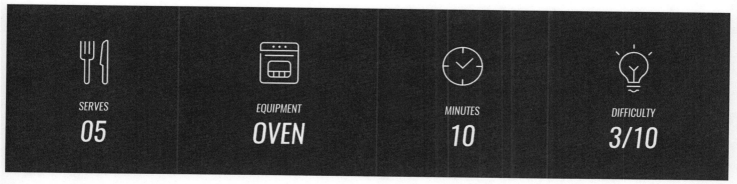

SERVES	EQUIPMENT	MINUTES	DIFFICULTY
05	OVEN	10	3/10

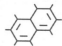

NUTRITIONAL INFORMATION PER ROLL:

245 CALORIES | 02 G CARBS | 20 G FAT | 12 G PROTEIN

INGREDIENTS

DRY INGREDIENTS

- **3.5 oz** almond meal *(100g)*
- **2 tbsp** psyllium husk powder
- **1 tsp** baking powder
- **2 tsp** sesame seeds
- **2 tsp** sunflower seeds
- **1 tsp** chia seeds
- **1/2 tsp** salt

WET INGREDIENTS

- **1 egg**
- **2** egg whites
- **1 tbsp** apple cider vinegar
- **3 tbsp** cooking coconut oil melted

PROCEDURE

Preheat oven to 350 F *(160 C)*.

In one bowl, mix all the dry ingredients together. In a separate bowl, mix together the wet ingredients with an electric beater.

Fold together the wet and dry ingredients. Slowly add some warm water until the mixture becomes slightly wet.

Roll into 5 balls, place on a tray and bake for 30 mins.

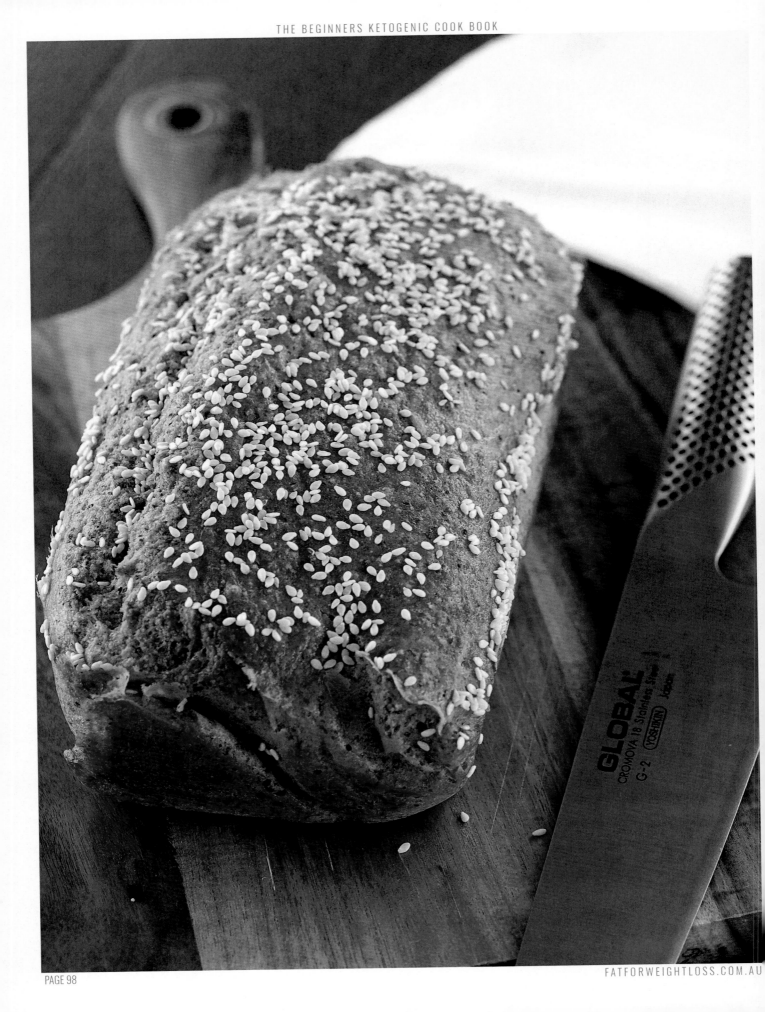

SEEDED KETO BREAD

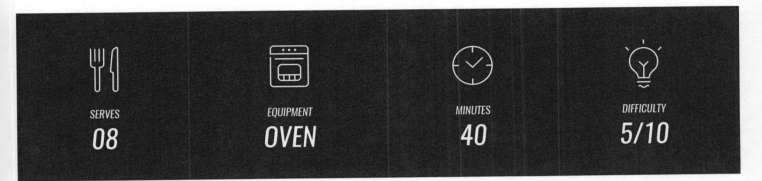

SERVES	EQUIPMENT	MINUTES	DIFFICULTY
08	OVEN	40	5/10

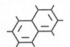

NUTRITIONAL INFORMATION PER 2 SLICES:

403 CALORIES | 03 G CARBS | 39 G FAT | 14 G PROTEIN

INGREDIENTS

- **1/2 cup** butter
- **2 tbsp** coconut oil
- **7 eggs**
- **1/4 cup** sunflower seeds
- **2 tbsp** chia seeds

- **3 tbsp** sesame seeds
- **1 tsp** baking powder
- **2 cups** almond flour
- **1/2 tsp** xanthan gum
- **1/2 tsp** salt

PROCEDURE

Preheat oven to 350F *(160C)*.

Put the eggs into a bowl and beat for 1 - 2 mins on high, Add the Xanthan gum and continue beating. Add coconut oil and melted butter to eggs, continue beating.

Add remaining ingredients except for sesame seeds.

Will become quite thick.

Scrape into a loaf pan lined with baking paper. Place sesame seeds on top.

Bake for 40 minutes. *(Remove once a skewer comes out of the middle clean).*

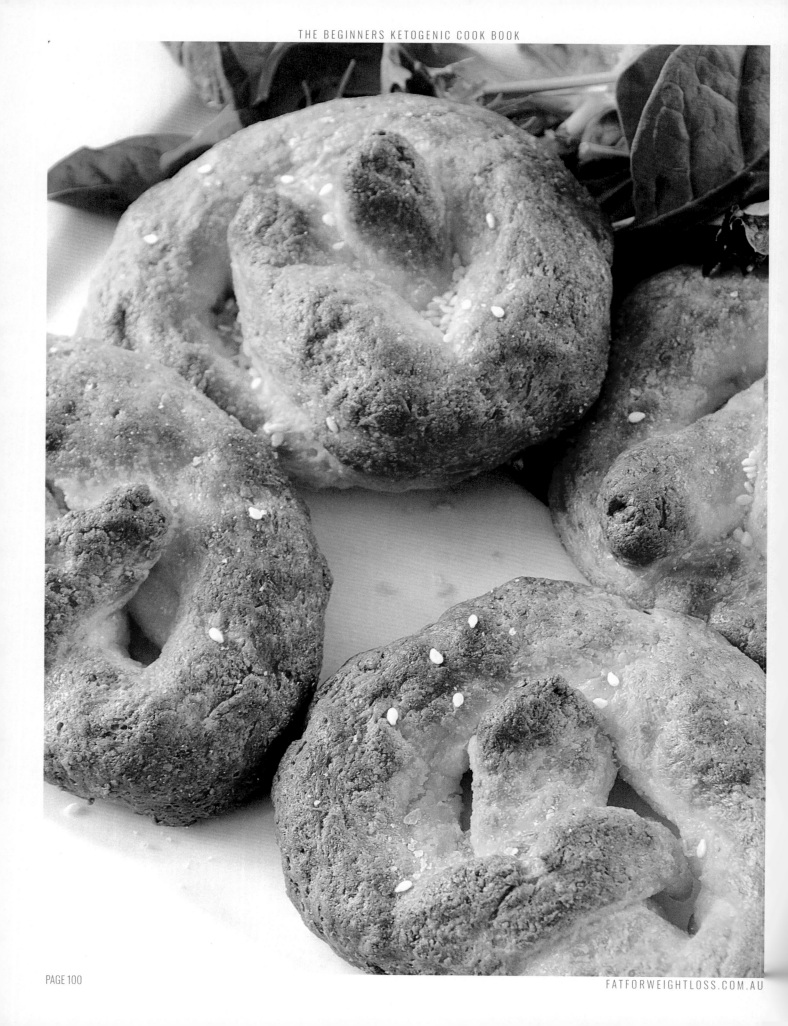

PRETZELS

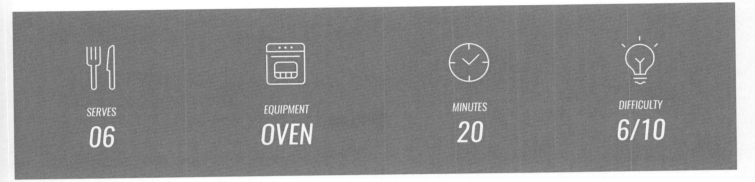

SERVES
06

EQUIPMENT
OVEN

MINUTES
20

DIFFICULTY
6/10

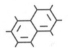

NUTRITIONAL INFORMATION:

209 CALORIES | 02 G CARBS | 18 G FAT | 11 G PROTEIN

INGREDIENTS

- **1.5 cups** mozzarella cheese
- **2 tbsp** cream cheese
- **3/4 cups** almond flour
- **1 tsp** xanthan gum

- **1 egg**
- **1 tsp** dried yeast
- **1 tbsp** warm water
- **1 tbsp** butter

PROCEDURE

Mix the cheese together into a microwave safe bowl, and heat on high in 30 second increments until the mixture is melted just enough to be able to bind completely. *(this should be about 1.5 mins).*

In a small cup, put the warm water and yeast together and let it sit for 3 mins to activate.

Mix the almond flour, egg and xanthium gum together in a bowl. I used an electric mixer for this.

Add the yeast and the water and mix together. Add the cheese and kneed the dough together with your hands.

Split into 4 balls, and roll out into long thin rolls.

Shape into pretzel round formations and place onto a baking tray. Cover with melted butter and bake in the oven at 200 degrees Celsius for 15 mins.

BREAD ROLLS

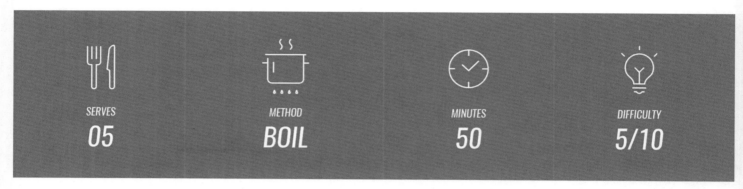

SERVES	METHOD	MINUTES	DIFFICULTY
05	BOIL	50	5/10

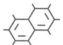

NUTRITIONAL INFORMATION PER ROLL:

735 CALORIES | 05 G CARBS | 13 G FAT | 12 G PROTEIN

INGREDIENTS

- **1 cup** almond meal
- **1/4 cup** golden flax seed meal
- **5 tbsp** psyllium husk powder
- **3 egg whites**

- **2 tbsp** apple cider vinegar
- **2 tsp** baking soda
- **1 tsp** salt
- **1 cup** boiling water

PROCEDURE

Preheat the oven to 375 F *(180C)*.

Get 2 mixing bowls, Both medium *(or 1 medium, 1 large)*. In medium sided mixing bowl, mix together all the dry ingredients *(Almond Flour, Golden Flax Seed Meal, Baking Soda, Salt and Psyllium Husk Powder)*.

Pro tip – If you don't have golden flax seed meal, you can use normal flaxseeds as well. I used a cheap electric coffee grinder to pulse the seeds down to a meal consistency.

In the second bowl, add the egg whites and beat them with an electric beater. Slowly add the apple cider vinegar once the egg whites become fluffy.

Next, combine the eggs with the dry ingredients.

Slowly add the hot water until the mixture starts to form a dough.

Split the dough into 5 pieces and roll into balls. Place on a tray lined with parchment paper *(baking paper)* and cook for approximately 50 mins.

BAGUETTE

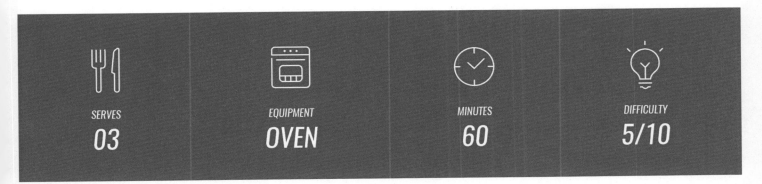

SERVES	EQUIPMENT	MINUTES	DIFFICULTY
03	OVEN	60	5/10

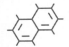

NUTRITIONAL INFORMATION:

192 CALORIES | 05 G CARBS | 10 G FAT | 11 G PROTEIN

INGREDIENTS

DRY INGREDIENTS

- **1/3 cup** almond flour *90g / 3 oz*
- **1/4 cup** psyllium husk powder *20g / 0.7 oz*
- **1/3 cup** coconut flour *40g / 1.4 oz*
- **1/2 tsp** baking soda
- **1 tsp** salt
- **1 tsp** xanthan gum

WET INGREDIENTS

- **3** Egg Whites
- **1** Whole Egg
- **1/4 cup** low-fat butter-milk *60g / 2.1 oz*
- **2 tbsp** apple cider vinegar *30ml / 1 floz*
- **1/3 cup** warm water *80ml / 2.7 floz*

PROCEDURE

Preheat the oven to 180 C / 360 F. Mix all of the dry ingredients together into a bowl.

In a different bowl, mix the butter-milk, egg whites and eggs together with an electric beater.

Add the egg mixture to the dry ingredients and mix well using the same mixer until the dough is relatively thick. Add vinegar and lukewarm water and process until well combined.

Using a spoon, scoop out sections and make a long baguette looking roll. You should be able to join together the different sections with your fingers.

Place in the oven and cook for 10 minutes, then reduce the heat to 160 C / 320 F and cook for another 30 - 40 mins. Cut and serve with Olive Oil and Balsamic!

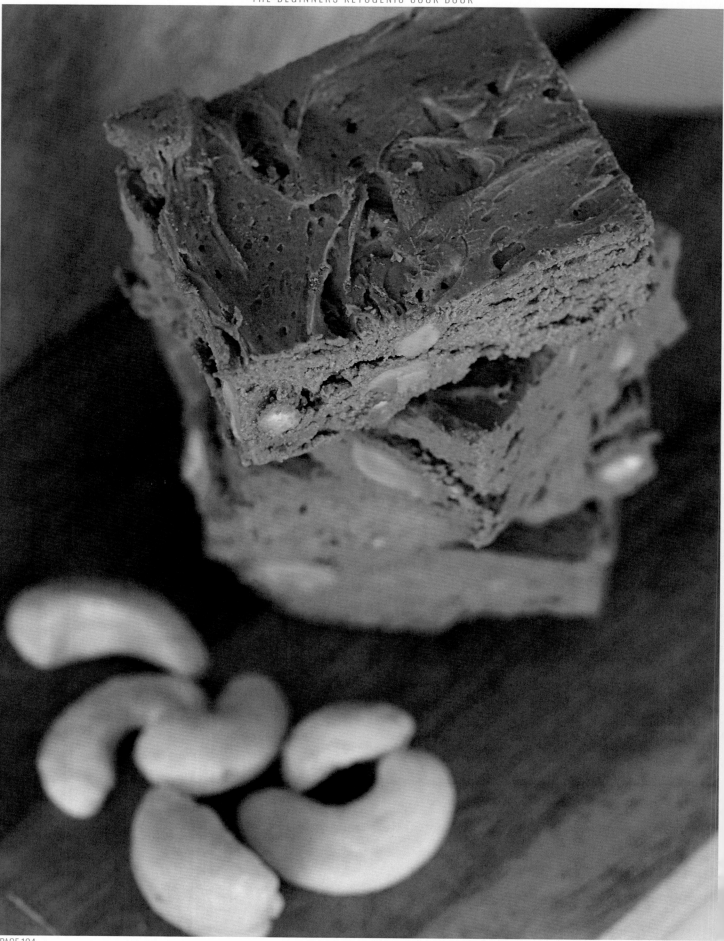

CHOCOLATE AND CASHEW FUDGE

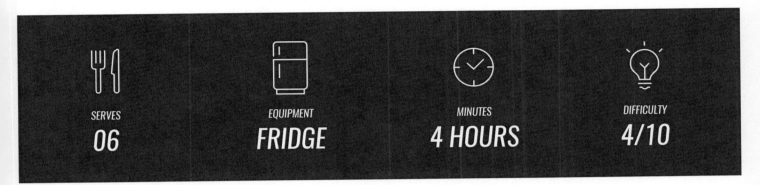

SERVES	EQUIPMENT	MINUTES	DIFFICULTY
06	FRIDGE	4 HOURS	4/10

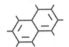

NUTRITIONAL INFORMATION:

233 CALORIES | **03 G CARBS** | **24 G FAT** | **03 G PROTEIN**

INGREDIENTS

- **1/2 cup** cream cheese (*120g / 4.2oz softened*)
- **1/2 cup** butter (*120g / 4.2oz softened*)
- **3 tbsp** unsweetened cocoa powder

- **2 tbsp** natvia (*or erythritol*)
- **1 tsp** vanilla extract
- **1.5 oz** cashews (*chopped 40g*)

PROCEDURE

Mix together the cream cheese and butter with an electric mixer.

Add the unsweetened cocoa powder, Natvia and vanilla extract. Mix until well combined and no lumps are present.

Add the cashews and continue mixing.

Place the mixture in a tray with baking paper. Place in the fridge for 4 hours to set.

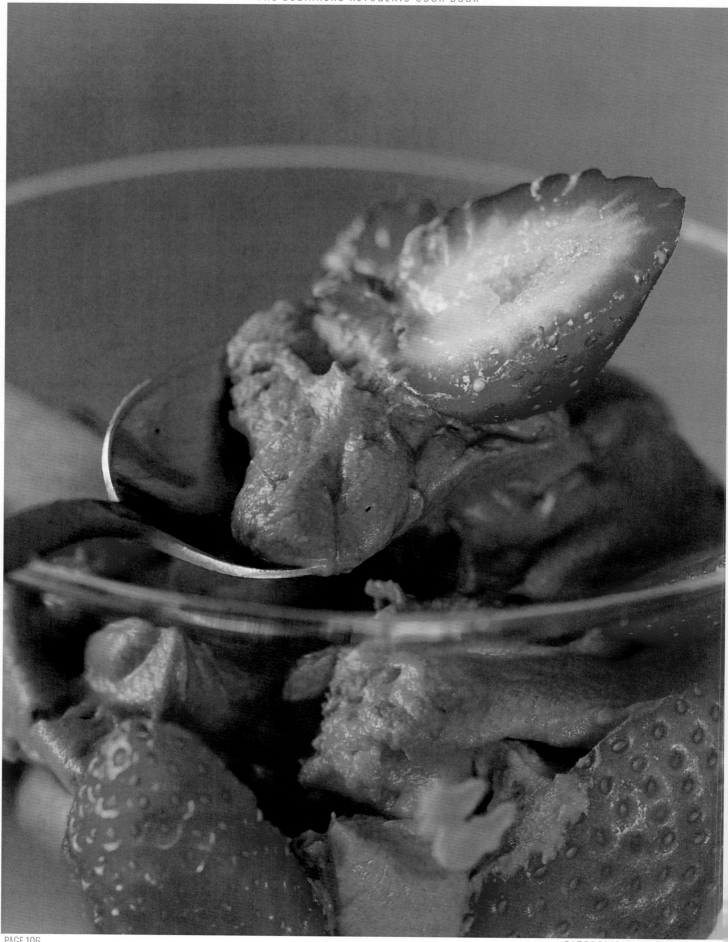

CHOCOLATE MOUSE

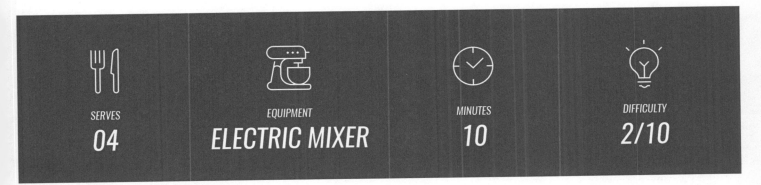

SERVES	EQUIPMENT	MINUTES	DIFFICULTY
04	ELECTRIC MIXER	10	2/10

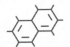

NUTRITIONAL INFORMATION:

292 CALORIES | **05 G CARBS** | **29 G FAT** | **05 G PROTEIN**

INGREDIENTS

- **8 oz** cream cheese (*250g*)
- **1/4 cup** cocoa powder unsweetened
- **1/2** large avocado, pitted

- **1/8 tsp** vanilla extract
- **3 tbsp** erythritol
- **1/4 cup** heavy whipping cream

PROCEDURE

Beat the cream cheese with an electric mixer.

Slowly add the avocado, cocoa powder, vanilla extract and erythritol until smooth. This should take around 5 mins.

In a separate mixing bowl, whip the heavy cream until stiff peaks form.

Place the whipped cream in the chocolate mixture and gently fold.

Place the chocolate mousse in a piping bag (*or Ziploc bag and cut the corner*) and press into cups.

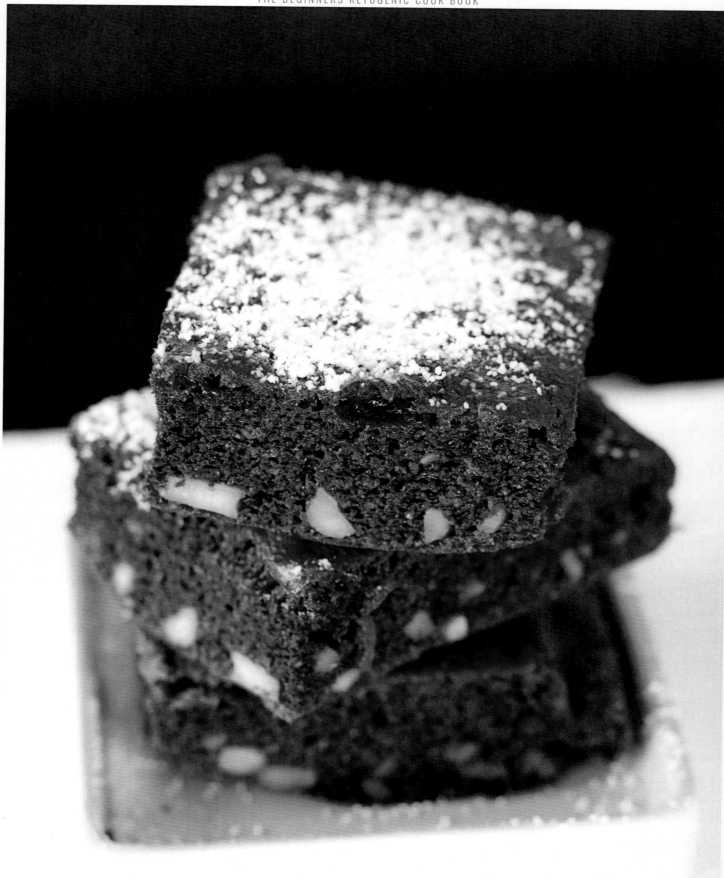

FUDGE BROWNIES

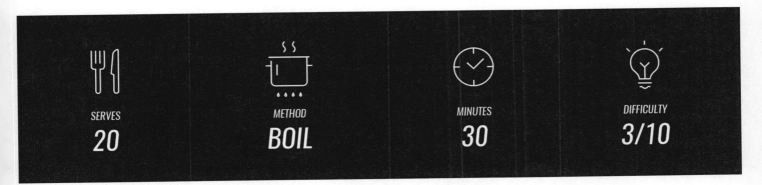

SERVES
20

METHOD
BOIL

MINUTES
30

DIFFICULTY
3/10

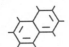 NUTRITIONAL INFORMATION PER BROWNIE:

112 CALORIES | 03 G CARBS | 11 G FAT | 03 G PROTEIN

INGREDIENTS

- **2.5 oz** almond flour (*75g*)
- **1/2 cup** butter (*unsalted 4 oz / 115g*)
- **6 oz** 80% dark chocolate (*170g*)
- **1/2 cup** natvia (*stevia or erythritol*)
- **4 eggs**

- **1/2 tsp** vanilla extract
- **1/2 tsp** baking powder
- **1 oz** cashews (*30 g*)
- **1** pinch salt

PROCEDURE

Preheat the oven to 320°F (*160°C*) line 9 x 9-in baking pan with baking paper.

Melt butter and chocolate in a microwave for 90 seconds. Set aside to cool.

Using a hand electric mixer, mix together the eggs, natvia (*stevia*), vanilla extract, and salt. Mix for around 3 minutes.

Then mix in the slightly cooled chocolate with the egg mixture until combined.

In a small bowl, stir together almond flour and baking powder.

Eventually add this into the chocolate egg mixture.

Put the mixture into the prepared baking pan Sprinkle with crushed cashews. You don't have to use cashews, you can use any nuts you like.

Put in the oven and bake for 25 - 30 minutes (*the less the fudgier*).

When a toothpick is inserted in the centre, it should still come out a little fudgy. This is perfect!

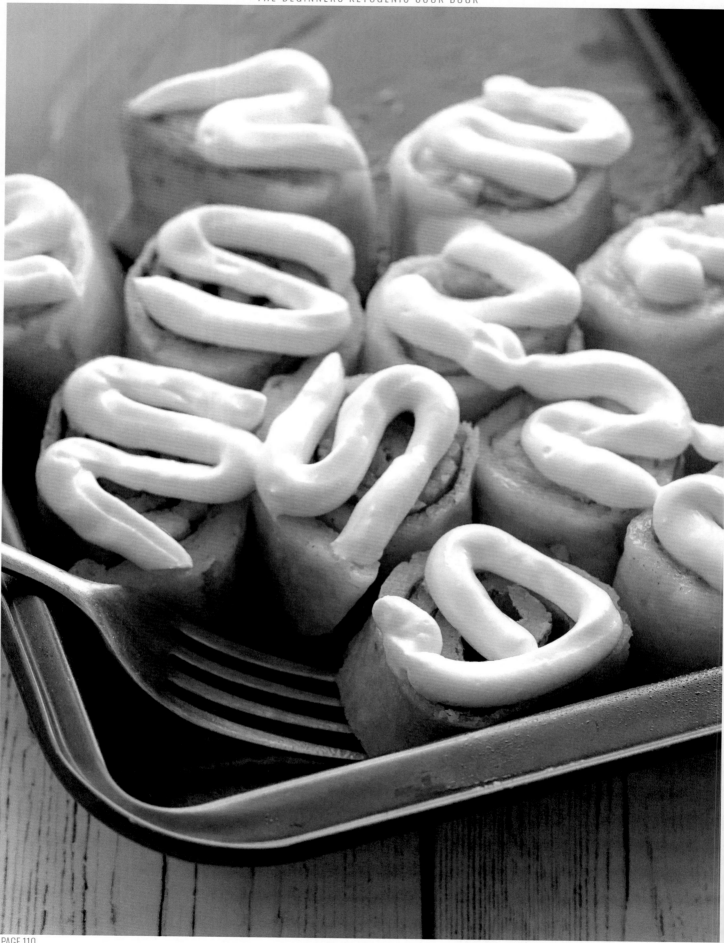

CINNAMON SCROLLS

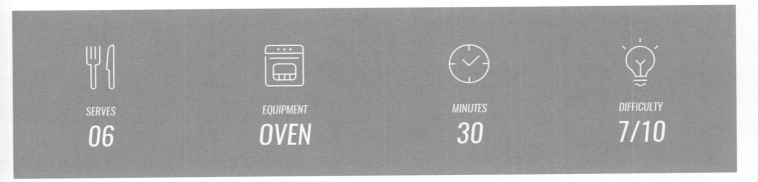

SERVES	EQUIPMENT	MINUTES	DIFFICULTY
06	OVEN	30	7/10

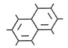

NUTRITIONAL INFORMATION:

307 CALORIES | 04 G CARBS | 25 G FAT | 06 G PROTEIN

INGREDIENTS

BASE
- **1.5 cups** mozzarella cheese
- **2 tbsp** cream cheese
- **1** egg
- **3/4 cups** almond flour
- **1 tbsp** erythritol

CINNAMON INSIDE
- **1 tbsp** erythritol
- **1 tsp** cinnamon
- **1 tbsp** warm water

ICING
- **1 tbsp** cream cheese
- **1 tbsp** heavy cream
- **1 tbsp** erythritol

PROCEDURE

Mix the cheese together into a microwave safe bowl, and heat on high in 30 second increments until the mixture is melted just enough to be able to bind completely. *(this should be about 1.5 mins).*

Mix in the stevia, egg, almond flour. Put in between two sheets of parchment paper and roll out into a rectangle.

Mix the stevia, cinnamon and water in a small cup and spread over the rolled out cheese mixture.

Begin from one side, and roll the scrolls into one long roll. Cut into 2 finger lengths and place onto a baking tray. Put in the oven at 375F *(180C)* for 10 mins.

Mix the cream cheese, cream and stevia together and but it into a plastic bag. Cut the corner off and pipe over the cinnamon scrolls.

Enjoy!

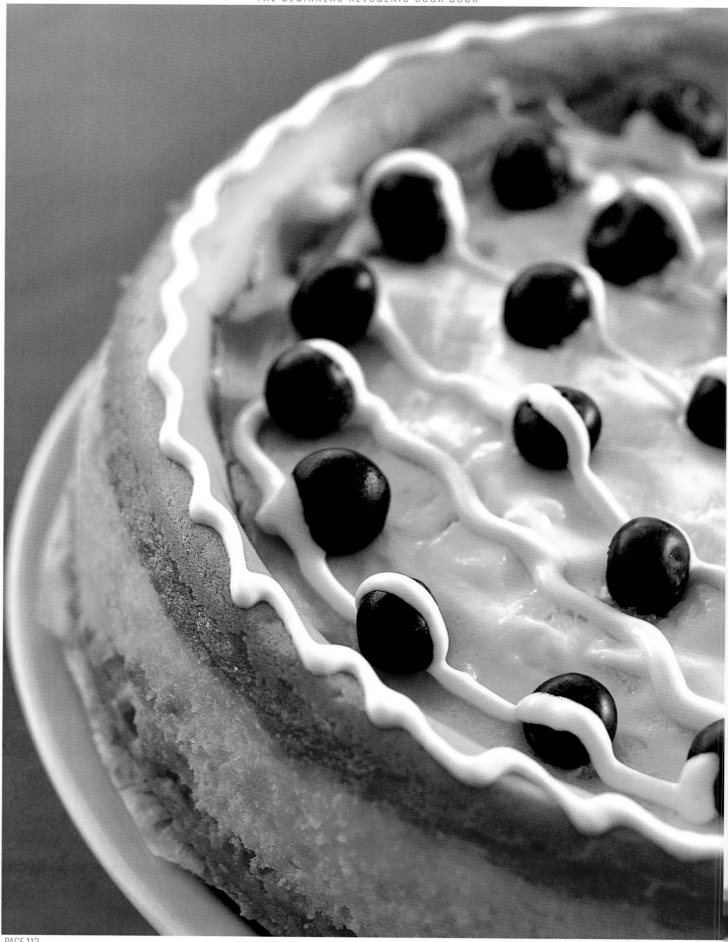

NEW YORK BAKED CHEESECAKE

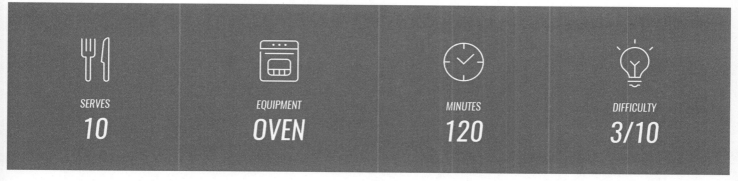

SERVES	EQUIPMENT	MINUTES	DIFFICULTY
10	**OVEN**	**120**	**3/10**

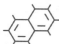

NUTRITIONAL INFORMATION PER SLICE:

305 CALORIES | 05 G CARBS | 27 G FAT | 08 G PROTEIN

INGREDIENTS

BASE
- **1/2 cups** almond flour
- **1/2 cups** coconut flour
- **1/4 cups** shredded coconut
- **1/2 cups** butter

CHEESE CAKE FILLING
- **2 cups** cream cheese
- **3/4 cups** sour cream
- **1/4 cups** erythritol
- **3** whole large eggs

- **1 tbsp** vanilla essence
- **1 tsp** lemon zest

PROCEDURE

Add all the base ingredients into a bowl, melt the butter in the microwave for 30 seconds and mix together in a bowl.

In a cake tin, line the inside with baking paper and press the base mixture into the bottom of the tin. I usually press it just to the bottom because the sides become too thin.

Place the tin in the fridge and continue to follow the steps.

Turn the oven on and select 140 degrees C (*280 F*) if fan forced, otherwise 160 degrees (*320 F*).

In a mixing bowl, add the cream cheese and the sour cream together, along with the vanilla essence and the lemon zest.

Add 1 Egg to the bowl and begin to mix together (*I use electric beaters to get a good consistency*). As the mixture begins to mix slightly, add another egg and continue to mix. Add the last egg and continue to mix.

Take the base out of the fridge and fill the tin with the cheese mixture. Put into the oven and bake for 45 - 50 mins. Check the cheesecake by pushing a spike into the middle. If it comes out clean then the cake is ready.

Leave the oven slight open and leave the cake in the oven for another 30 mins to cool slowly. Put in the fridge for another 60 mins and enjoy!

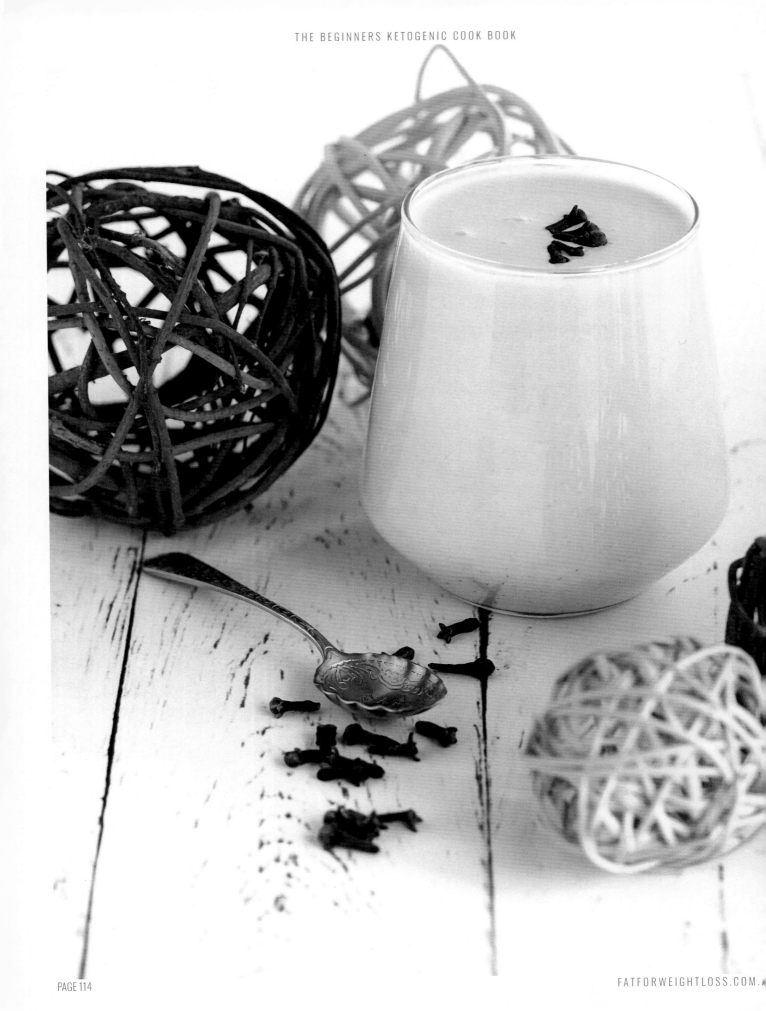

EGG NOG

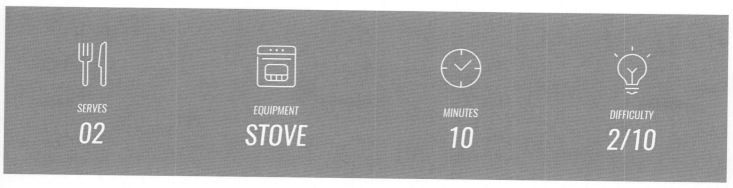

SERVES
02

EQUIPMENT
STOVE

MINUTES
10

DIFFICULTY
2/10

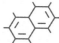

NUTRITIONAL INFORMATION PER SERVING:

660 CALORIES | **05 G CARBS** | **57 G FAT** | **07 G PROTEIN**

INGREDIENTS

- **1 cup** coconut milk
- **1 tsp** nutmeg ground
- **4** cloves
- **1 tsp** vanilla extract

- **3** egg yolks
- **1 cup** heavy cream
- **2.5 oz** rum *(80 ml)*
- **2 tbsp** stevia *(natvia)*

PROCEDURE

Mix together on low heat the coconut milk, cloves and nutmeg in a pot on the stove. Mix together the egg yolks and stevia in a bowl. Add the vanilla essence into the pan.

Once the coconut milk has become hot, mix the egg yolks in and continue to stir for 3 mins until the mixture becomes thick, but not gluggy.

Strain the cloves out from the mixture and serve into a cup, pour the cream and rum into the cup afterwards and mix through as little or as much as you like!

Or put it in the fridge for a delicious cold eggnog *(the contents still stay mixed together)*.

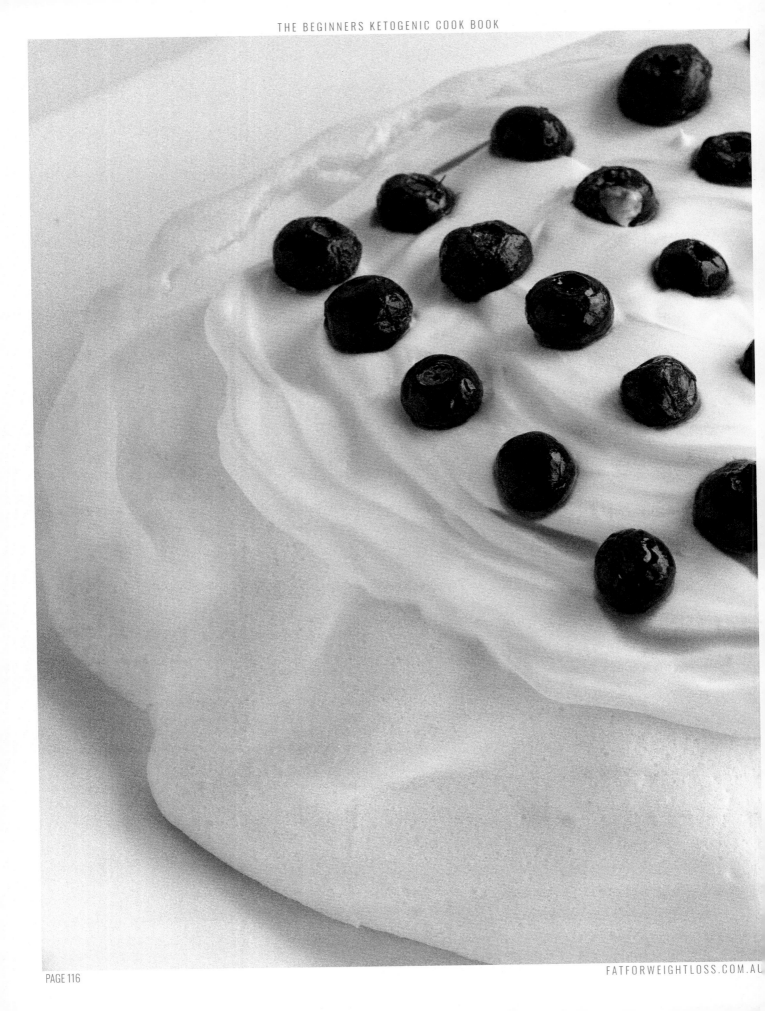

MERINGUE (PAVLOVA)

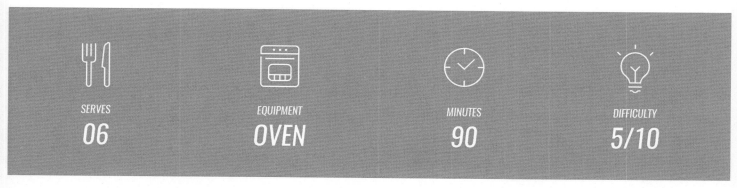

SERVES	EQUIPMENT	MINUTES	DIFFICULTY
06	OVEN	90	5/10

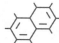

NUTRITIONAL INFORMATION:

257 CALORIES | **04 G CARBS** | **15 G FAT** | **05 G PROTEIN**

INGREDIENTS

- **6** egg whites
- **1/2 cups** sugar substitute
- **1 tsp** white vinegar
- **1 tsp** vanilla essence

- **10 fl oz** double cream (*300ml*)
- **1/2** punnet blueberries
- **2 tsp** almond flour

PROCEDURE

Preheat the oven to 245F (*120 C*). Separate the egg whites into a mixing bowl. Beat with a mixer until peaks begin to form. Slowly add in the stevia whilst beating. Beat for and extra 1 min. Add in the vinegar, flour and vanilla and beat for another 1 min.

Place aluminum foil onto a baking tray and outline the size of a large dinner plate. Spoon the fluffy mixture into the circle and add some of your own mega awesome artwork to the fluffy outsides with a spoon.

Place in the oven for 1 hour 30 mins.

Once the timer has gone off, Leave the door open and let it cool down to room temperature. Place onto a plate and top with double cream (*you can whip this slightly if you like*) and top with the blueberries.

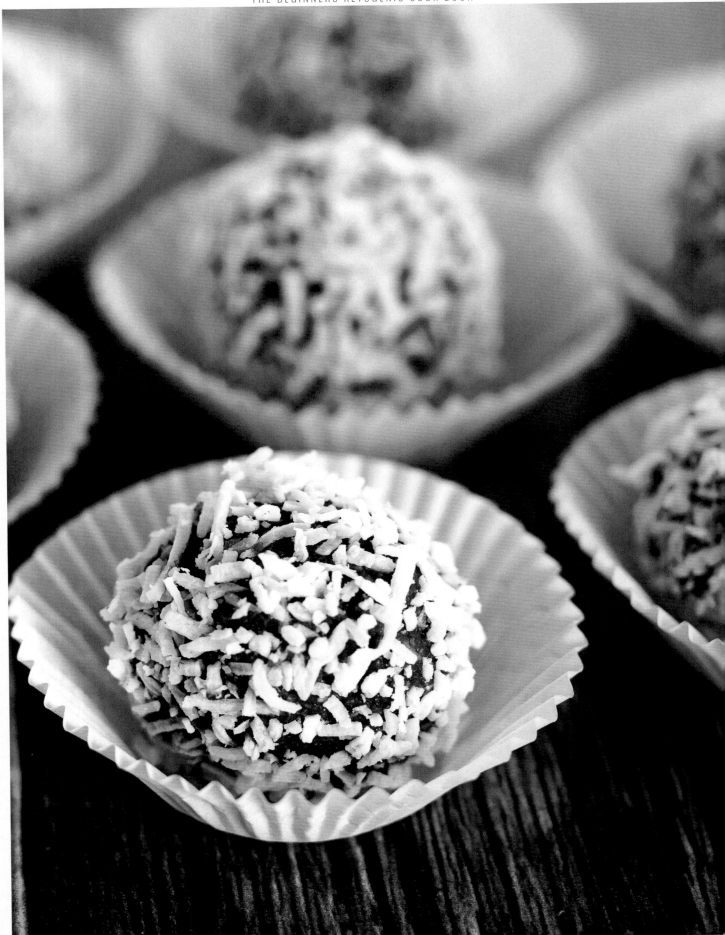

RUM BALLS (FAT BOMBS)

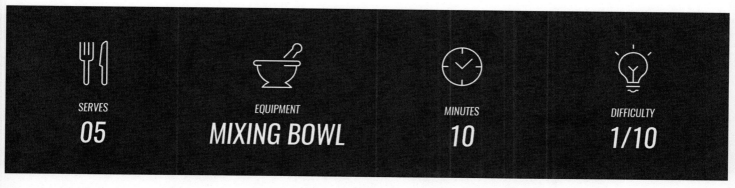

SERVES
05

EQUIPMENT
MIXING BOWL

MINUTES
10

DIFFICULTY
1/10

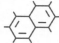 NUTRITIONAL INFORMATION:

290 CALORIES | **03 G CARBS** | **25 G FAT** | **06 G PROTEIN**

INGREDIENTS

- **1/4 cups** cocoa powder
- **1/4 cups** coconut oil
- **1/4 cups** almond flour
- **2 tbsp** heavy cream

- **1/2 cups** shredded coconut
- **2 tsp** stevia
- **60 ml** rum

PROCEDURE

Mix all the ingredients together into a bowl. Combine until sticky. Depending on the weather, if it gets to sloppy, just add some more almond flour to the mix.

Roll into balls and roll in some extra shredded coconut. (*I blended my shredded coconut in the nutri-bullet so it was smaller shreds*). Let the disco overwhelm you as you point to the sky, then point to the floor whilst making these ones!

Refrigerate on a plate and enjoy!

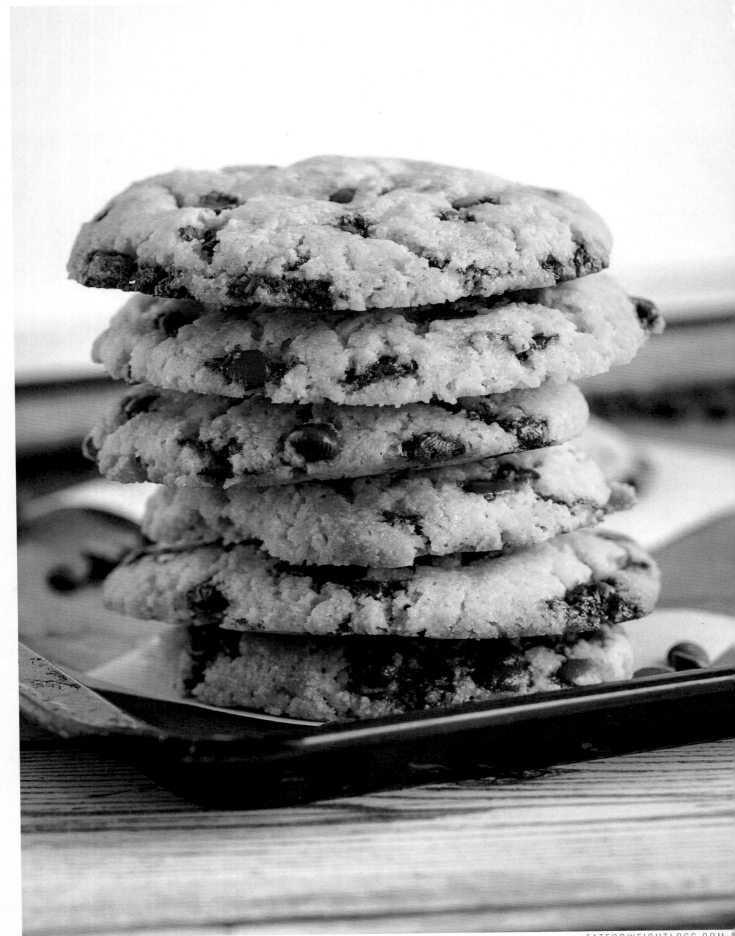

CHOCOLATE CHIP COOKIES

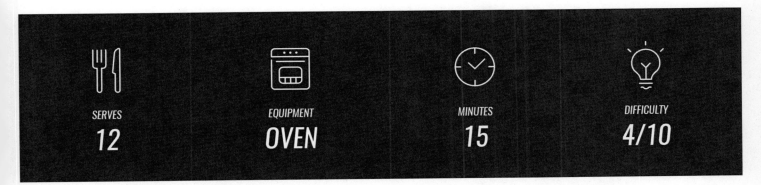

SERVES
12

EQUIPMENT
OVEN

MINUTES
15

DIFFICULTY
4/10

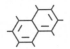

NUTRITIONAL INFORMATION PER COOKIE:

168 CALORIES | **02 G CARBS** | **17 G FAT** | **04 G PROTEIN**

INGREDIENTS

- **1 1/2 cups** almond flour
- **1/2 cup** salted butter
- **3/4 cup** erythritol
- **1 tsp** vanilla extract

- **1/2 tsp** baking powder
- **1/4 tsp** salt
- **1/2 tsp** xanathan gum
- **3/4 cup** sugar free chocolate chips

PROCEDURE

Preheat your oven to 180C *(355 F)*.

Zap the butter for 30 seconds to melt, but it shouldn't be hot.

Place the butter into a mixing bowl and beat with the natvia. Add the vanilla and egg, mix on low for another 15 seconds exactly.

Add the almond flour, xanthan gum, baking powder and salt. Mix until well combined.

Press the dough together and remove from the bowl.

Combine the chocolate chips into the dough with your hands.

Roll the dough to Make 12 balls and place on a baking tray. Bake for 10 mins.

Let them cool, and serve. Keep in an airtight container.

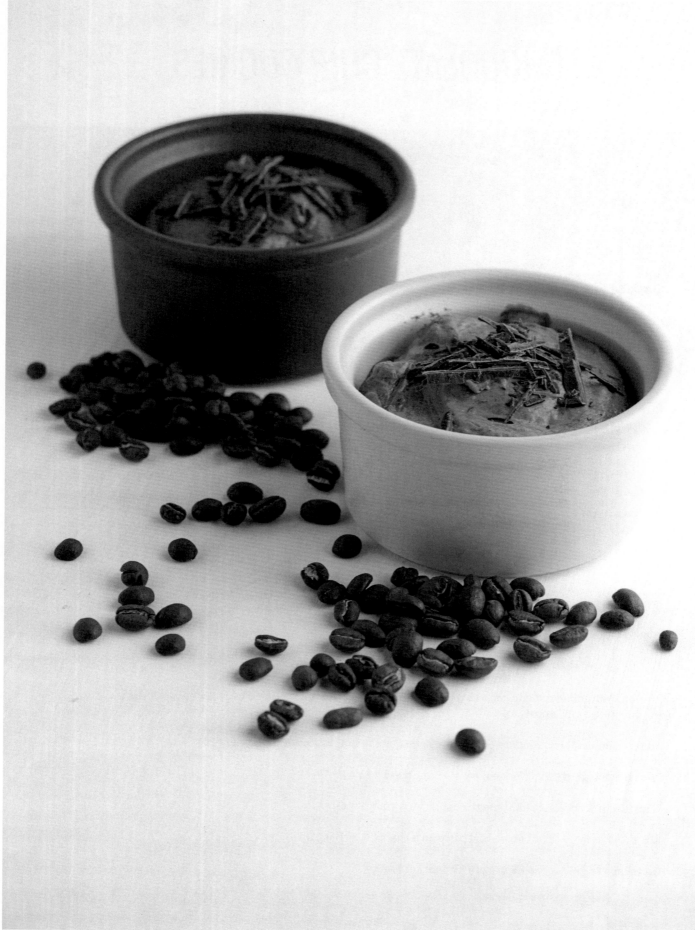

CHOCOLATE COFFEE PUDDING

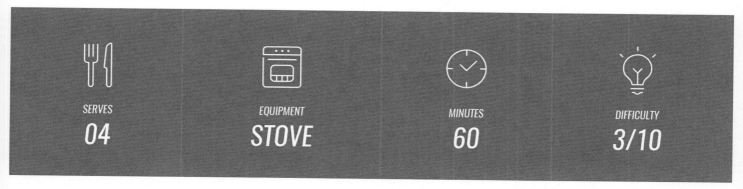

SERVES
04

EQUIPMENT
STOVE

MINUTES
60

DIFFICULTY
3/10

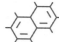 NUTRITIONAL INFORMATION PER SERVING:

345 CALORIES | **05 G CARBS** | **35 G FAT** | **04 G PROTEIN**

INGREDIENTS

- **1/2 cup** unsweetened cocoa
- **1/2 cup** sugar substitute
- **1 oz** shot espresso *(30 ml)*
- **1/2 tsp** xanthan gum
- **1 ½ cups** heavy whipping cream

PROCEDURE

In a small saucepan, slowly heat up the heavy cream whilst adding the cocoa, expresso, and the sugar substitute.

Once the cocoa and sugar has mixed in, add the xanthan gum and slowly bring to simmer.

Once the mixture starts to become thick, remove from the heat, place into ramekins *(or bowls)* and chill for 1 hour.

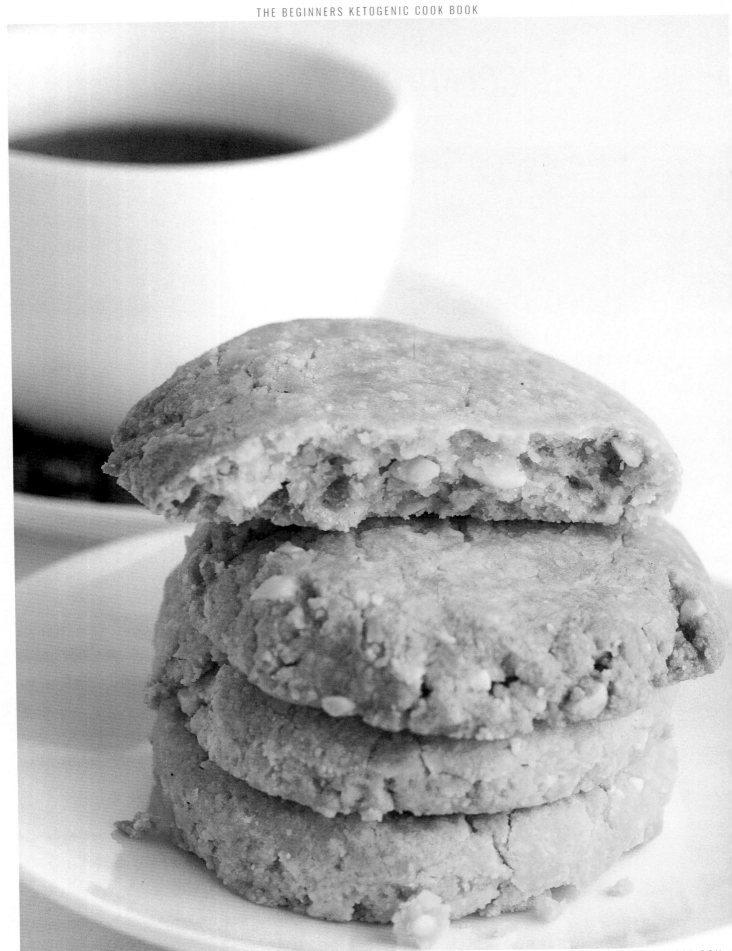

PEANUT BUTTER COOKIES

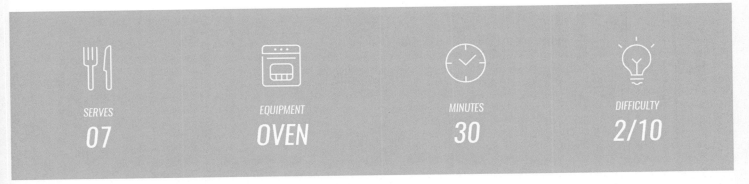

SERVES	EQUIPMENT	MINUTES	DIFFICULTY
07	OVEN	30	2/10

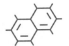

NUTRITIONAL INFORMATION PER COOKIE:

215 CALORIES | **05 G CARBS** | **19 G FAT** | **08 G PROTEIN**

INGREDIENTS

- **1 cup** no sugar peanut butter
- **2/3 cup** sugar substitute
- **1** large egg
- **1/2 tsp** vanilla extract
- **1/2 tsp** salt

PROCEDURE

Preheat oven to 350F (*180C*). Mix all of the ingredients in a large bowl until well combined.

Roll them into 7 balls and squash flat with a fork (*alternatively, use the bottom of a large muffin tin and press the balls into the bottom of the pans to form perfect circles without breaking bits*).

Bake for 15 – 20 mins until they start to turn slightly brown.

Cool on a baking tray for 20 mins and enjoy!

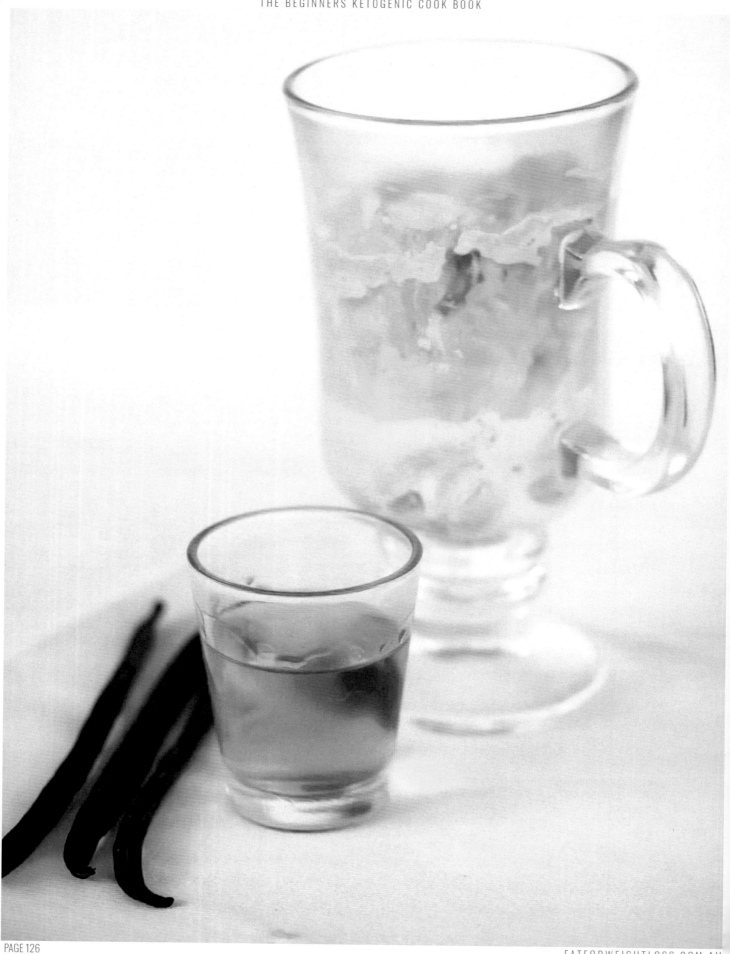

VANILLA RUM MUG CAKE

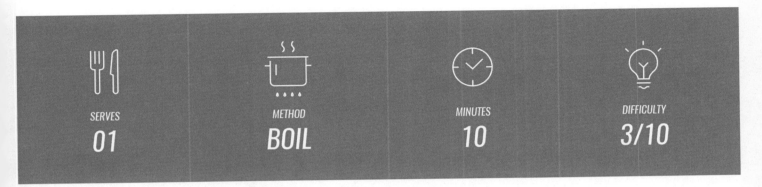

SERVES
01

METHOD
BOIL

MINUTES
10

DIFFICULTY
3/10

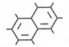

NUTRITIONAL INFORMATION:

398 CALORIES | **04 G CARBS** | **29 G FAT** | **10 G PROTEIN**

INGREDIENTS

- **1** egg
- **2 tbsp** butter
- **2 tbsp** almond meal
- **1 tbsp** heavy cream

- **1 tbsp** sugar substitute
- **1/2 tsp** baking powder
- **1 tsp** vanilla extract
- **1 oz** rum *(or 1 tsp rum extract)*

PROCEDURE

Mix all ingredients except for the cream together in a mug.

Microwave on high for 90 seconds.

Cover with cream and enjoy!

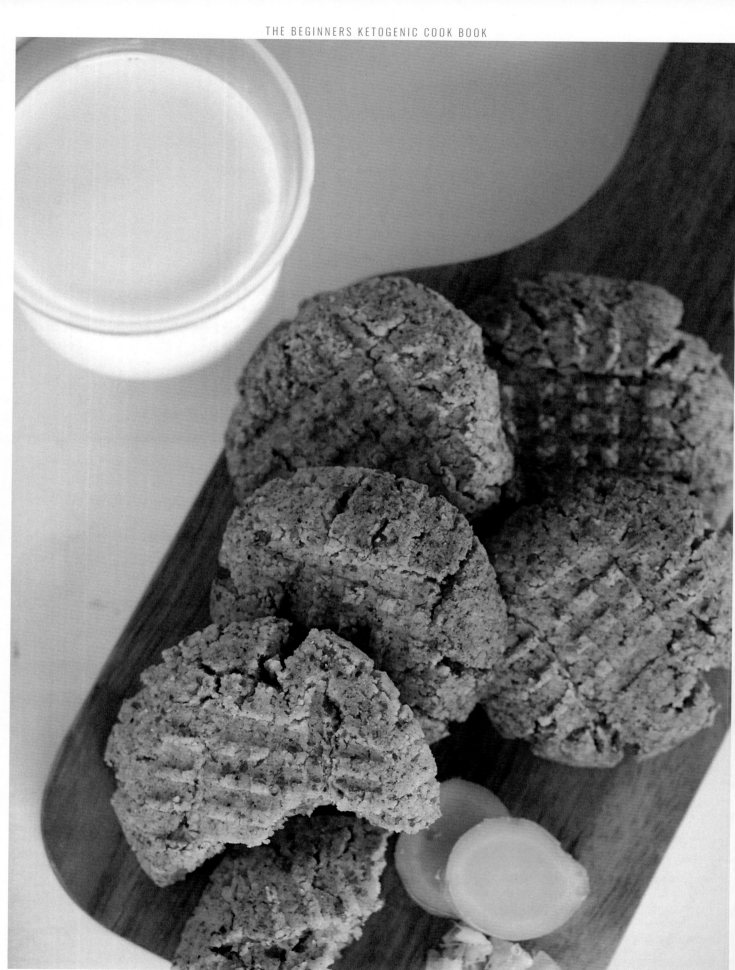

GINGER AND CLOVE COOKIES

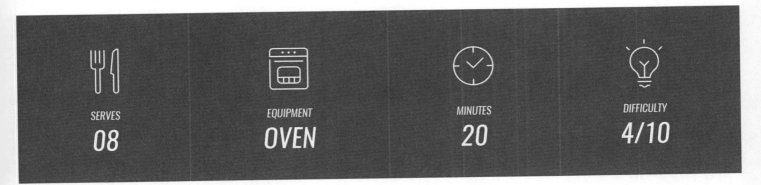

SERVES	EQUIPMENT	MINUTES	DIFFICULTY
08	OVEN	20	4/10

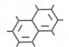

NUTRITIONAL INFORMATION:

205 CALORIES | **03 G CARBS** | **19 G FAT** | **06 G PROTEIN**

INGREDIENTS

- **1 ¾ cups** almond flour
- **3 tbsp** sugar substitute
- **2 tsp** ginger ground
- **1/4 tsp** cloves ground
- **1 tsp** cinnamon ground

- **1/4 tsp** nutmeg ground
- **1/4 cup** butter unsalted
- **1** egg
- **1 tsp** vanilla extract
- **1/4 tsp** salt

PROCEDURE

Pre heat the oven to 355 F (*180 C*). Mix all the dry ingredients together into a bowl.

Mix all the wet ingredients together in with the dry ingredients. Roll the mixture into 8 balls and press flat with a fork.

Place baking paper onto a baking tray and place the cookies in the oven for 12-15 mins or until slightly brown on top. Keep in an airtight container.

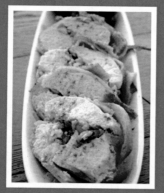
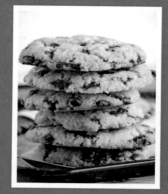
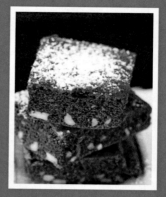
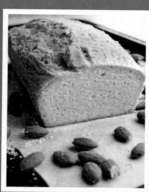
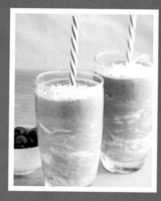
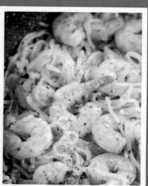

The Beginner's
KETOGENIC COOKBOOK

You might not believe weight loss without exercise is possible. You probably don't believe it's possible to perform in a healthier way during exercise. You may not think it's possible to build muscle whilst restricting carbohydrates, and most of all, what could be healthy about increasing your fat intake?

This book explains the ketogenic diet in very simple terms. The basic idea of the ketogenic diet is focused on re-teaching your own body to turn to fat for energy instead of carbohydrates, burning fat for energy as it needs to.

Excess carbohydrates turn to fat in the body anyway, so doesn't it make sense to train your body to burn fat if you want to lose fat?

There are many benefits of eating a ketogenic diet. Effortless weight loss increased brain clarity and elimination of many common diseases such as Epilepsy, Diabetes, Polycystic Ovary Syndrome (PCOS), Irritable Bowel Syndrome (IBS), GERD, heartburn and Non-alcoholic fatty liver disease (NAFLD).

Aaron is a low carb ketogenic food blogger, photographer, and enthusiast with experience in nutritional therapy and advanced sports exercise nutrition. This cookbook aims to help you through your keto journey by sharing simple keto recipes, low carb recipes and carbohydrate replacements for everyday meals. This book puts your health first.

Made in the USA
Lexington, KY
05 November 2018